The International Behavioura

STUDIES ON PSYCHOSIS

TAVISTOCK

The International Behavioural and Social Sciences Library

MENTAL HEALTH
In 8 Volumes

STUDIES ON PSYCHOSIS

Descriptive, Psycho-Analytic and Psychological Aspects

THOMAS FREEMAN
WITH JOHN L CAMERON AND
ANDREW McGHIE

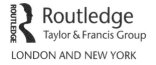

LONDON AND NEW YORK

First published in 1965 by
Tavistock Publications Limited

Published in 2001 by
Routledge
2 Park Square, Milton Park, Abingdon, Oxfordshire OX14 4RN
711 Third Avenue, New York, NY 10017

First issued in paperback 2014

Routledge is an imprint of the Taylor and Francis Group, an informa business

British Library Cataloguing in Publication Data
A CIP catalogue record for this book
is available from the British Library

Studies on Psychosis
ISBN 0-415-26449-9
Mental Health: 8 Volumes
ISBN 0-415-26511-8
The International Behavioural and Social Sciences Library
112 Volumes
ISBN 0-415-25670-4

ISBN 13: 978-1-138-87588-3 (pbk)
ISBN 13: 978-0-415-26449-5 (hbk)

Studies on Psychosis

DESCRIPTIVE, PSYCHO-ANALYTIC, AND
PSYCHOLOGICAL ASPECTS

THOMAS FREEMAN M.D., M.R.C.P.(Ed.), D.P.M.
The Lansdowne Clinic, Glasgow

with JOHN L. CAMERON M.B., B.Ch., D.P.M.
Chestnut Lodge Sanitarium, Rockville, U.S.A.

and ANDREW McGHIE M.A., Ph.D.
Director, Department of·Clinical Psychology, Royal Dundee Liff Hospital,
Hon. Lecturer in Psychology, Queen's College, Dundee

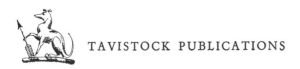 TAVISTOCK PUBLICATIONS

First published in 1965
by Tavistock Publications Limited
2 Park Square, Milton Park, Abingdon, Oxon, OX14 4RN
Set in 11 point Monotype Bembo, one point leaded
© Thomas Freeman 1965

Contents

Acknowledgements

The principal author wishes to acknowledge the assistance received from the Medical Research Council and the Henderson Research Scholarship in Mental Diseases. He is indebted to those colleagues with whom he has worked during the past twelve years. He would like to thank Dr W. T. McClatchey for permission to describe Case 18 in Chapter 7, Mr C. E. Gathercole for conducting psychological tests, and Miss C. Kerr and Miss C. McCormick for typing the manuscript. Finally he is grateful to many patients for their co-operation.

CHAPTER 1

Introduction

There is a growing awareness among psychiatrists, psycho-analysts, and psychologists that the isolationism which has existed between their separate disciplines must be swept away if advances are to be made in the understanding of mental illness. This isolationism, which at one time was necessary to allow each speciality to build up its concepts and methods of study, now acts as an obstacle to progress. It is to be hoped that this book will help to diminish the distance between the different disciplines by demonstrating the amount of common ground that exists between them in the field of the functional psychoses. Those who work with the concepts of two or more of these disciplines know how often a different terminology describes identical phenomena and identical hypotheses.

In order to fulfil the aim of this book, descriptive accounts of patients are given in detail throughout the succeeding chapters alongside psycho-analytic formulations. In Chapter 9 Dr McGhie gives an account of the experimental studies on which he has been engaged over the past five years. The results of these investigations into the defects of attention, immediate memory, and perception in the schizophrenias complement certain aspects of the clinical hypotheses developed in earlier chapters. Chapter 10, contributed by Dr J. L. Cameron, is concerned with the psycho-analytic treatment of the psychoses. In it he describes details of administrative technique and patient management and presents illustrations of the interaction that occurs between patient and physician during therapy.

In the first two decades of this century psycho-analysis evoked a new and exciting interest in the psychology of the psychoses. The effect of Freud's theory of schizophrenia and paranoia (1911) was to make psychiatrists take another look at the clinical phenomena that these conditions presented. The enthusiasm of some was only matched by the cynicism of others. Hopes of a psycho-analytic treatment for the schizophrenias were never encouraged by Freud and his immediate circle, but they flourished none the less. Thus, over the past forty years, many accounts have appeared in the literature of successful and unsuccessful attempts to apply the psycho-analytic method to cases of schizophrenia. Today the interest of those early years has all but vanished and many psychiatrists are inclined to regard the psycho-analytic approach to the psychoses as rather superfluous and of little value in either treatment or research. This judgement is generally made by those who are not psycho-analysts and by those who have not studied psycho-analytic theories and concepts. However, this argument alone cannot grant to psycho-analysis a place in the study and treatment of the psychoses. It is incumbent upon psycho-analysts to demonstrate how the theories and methods of psycho-analysis can be fruitfully employed in both research and therapy.

What has psycho-analysis to contribute to research in the psychoses? It can make two important contributions. First, it offers a technique whereby contact can be made with the patient thus enabling him to reveal his subjective experiences. Psycho-analytic technique makes allowances for the fact that it takes time – not necessarily years – before a patient can talk freely and without reserve. It also warns the clinician not to accept the patient's denials or reluctance to communicate as anything other than manifestations of his anxiety. Psycho-analysis is frequently misunderstood as being a technique of indoctrination. Be that as it may, psycho-analytic technique lays stress upon the psycho-analyst's refraining from impetuous interpretation until he has obtained a good relationship with the patient and amassed considerable detail about him.

This aspect of psycho-analytic method requires emphasis because, once a relationship has been established between patient and interviewer, psycho-analysis can be used as a technique for investigation. It is unnecessary to envisage psycho-analytic contact with a psychotic patient as one in which the psycho-analyst must give interpretations to the patient about his unconscious conflicts and phantasies. The clinical contact can be maintained by showing a friendly interest and only when necessary bringing out the patient's fears of the interview situation.

There are limits beyond which the method cannot penetrate because some patients refuse to talk. Fortunately there are many who will communicate freely if given the opportunity. It is unnecessary to 'indoctrinate' patients and it can be confidently maintained that the patient's utterances need not be seriously influenced by the investigator's interventions. The data obtained can be recorded in different ways. This in itself is a difficulty because in the end the material must be assessed subjectively by whoever is seeing the patient, and each clinician has his own criteria for a particular clinical concept.

The day has arrived when such concepts as flattening of affect and perplexity must be discarded. Clinicians must confine themselves to data that are less dependent upon the subjective impressions of the examiner. There are enough discrete and definable phenomena which the patient manifests and which are independent of the interviewer's subjective assessments. They can be recorded on tape or simply noted down. Rating scales are useful, too, but again the investigator must recognize that, even if all were agreed about the meaning of a particular clinical concept, the rating decided upon only provides inexact information about the patient's mental activity at that one minute in time. It should not be given the significance of a physical measurement which can be obtained from a laboratory in bodily disease.

Psycho-analysis has a second contribution to make in providing the investigator with a theory of mental illness that is closely integrated with its general theory of mental functioning. Psycho-analysis, apart from its therapeutic aspects, offers a developmental theory of mind with an emphasis upon the emergence of differentiated mental activity from a matrix of primitive, syncretic mental processes. Freud (1900) distinguished between two modes of mental functioning which operate in the healthy adult – the primary and secondary processes (see Chapter 2). The former is tied to the instinctual needs, whereas the latter, being independent of the drives, facilitates environmental adaptation. The secondary process can roughly be equated with Freud's ego concept (1923), which includes cognition and defence against the drives. It allows the drives a controlled expression and neutralizes the instinctual energy necessary for motivation. The concept of regression as employed in the psychoses means no more than that the primary-process mode of mental function obtains an ascendancy. There is much in common between this psycho-analytic theory and that of the genetic psychologists, who also look upon the psychoses as the outcome of a primitivization of mental function.

Psycho-analysis lays stress upon the connection between mental functioning and interpersonal relationships, and there is a good deal of clinical evidence to support this hypothesis. It is unjust to psycho-analysis to infer that this claim implies that interpersonal conflicts are the cause of psychotic illnesses. All that can be said is that in some instances changes in interpersonal relations are paralleled by changes in cognitive functions. This knowledge can be fruitfully employed in observing and studying patients, because it alerts the observer to phe-nomena he might otherwise ignore. The content of a patient's frag-mented and incoherent utterances might be entirely related to the interview situation and to the interviewer.

According to psycho-analytic theory, it is the endopsychic (uncon-scious) reaction to object relationships that initiates the pathological process. It is unnecessary here to go into the details of the content of such endopsychic complexes. It is sufficient to emphasize that the theory proposes that these unconscious complexes provoke anxiety and guilt – perhaps of a special kind – which in turn leads to the primitivization (regression) of the mental functioning. It is well known, for example, that the form and content of a patient's utterances will change as a result of affective influences. It is also known that a patient's capacity to attend and concentrate can easily be disturbed by the intrusion of misperceptions and hallucinations which are stimulated by a disturb-ance in object relationships.

There is still much to be gained from an examination of the relation-ship that exists between dreams and schizophrenic manifestations. The similarities between them have been commented upon by many authorities since Hughlings Jackson made his famous statement, reported by Ernest Jones, that once we can understand dreams we will understand psychosis. The dream is first and foremost a hallucinatory experience – at the same time it presents a form of mental functioning quite unlike what is encountered in the waking state. Images change in shape, they are condensed; either words are used inappropriately or new ones are invented. Temporal and spatial relationships no longer apply, and the laws of syntax are frequently in abeyance. Thought and perceptual processes operate in a manner quite unlike that of the waking state – particularly when sustained concentration of attention is required. It is also true that the content of many dreams is as logical and coherent as a fragment of waking life.

Rapaport (1951) has, among his many other important contributions, pointed out that the dream is a special state of consciousness (a cognitive organization) which can be compared with that of the day-dream, the hypnagogic state, and that which characterizes the state of attention and concentration. In each of these states thinking and perceiving have their own laws. It would seem as if the state of consciousness associated with the dream has an important similarity to that of certain psychotic illnesses. Under special conditions patients can be observed in whom a transition occurs from the cognitive organization necessary for sustained attention and verbal communication to the cognitive dysfunction that is the essence of the disorganization of thinking and perceiving characteristic of some of the schizophrenias.

The question remains as to whether or not all psychotic phenomena have a background of unconscious conflict or have a latent content in the same fashion as the dream. Some psycho-analysts would answer this question in the affirmative, proposing that in the schizophrenias the whole symptom complex is by way of being a defensive structure set up to protect a true or real self which has never been able to find an outlet because of the belief in its own and others' omnipotent destructiveness. This is a psycho-analytic hypothesis which can never be subjected to clinical or psychological testing because it is essentially a subjective interpretation of clinical data. Though it is true that all psycho-analytical hypotheses are based upon abstractions from clinical data, the decisive factor must always be how far the abstraction proceeds — the nearer the abstractions are to the phenomena themselves the more credible they become.

Much psychiatric research is currently undertaken by super-specialists. The descriptive psychiatrist studies phenomena — this approach is not so fashionable nowadays but it may be beginning to regain its former status and prestige. The psycho-analyst confines himself to the consulting-room and hoards away the rich clinical material which he obtains from his patients. He has not, in spite of the example of Schilder (1923) and others, recognized the value of discussing his data with colleagues in other psychiatric disciplines. This tendency is gradually being reversed, at least in the United States, and the process may eventually occur here. It is hoped that the present book will hasten this trend. Lastly, the psychologist works away with his tests and statistical methods, very often without sufficient clinical experience or detailed knowledge of patients he is dealing with and, worst of all, letting commonsense fly out of the window.

To many psychiatrists there appears to be an irreconcilable conflict between the clinical and inferential method of psycho-analysis and the direct, objective approach of clinical psychology. Thus far (see

Chapter 9) the results of psychological studies on the schizophrenias, for example, do not invalidate or clash with the basic psycho-analytic conception of the psychotic process (Freud, 1911). In a recent publication, Shakow has detailed a number of criteria, based upon experimental studies, which distinguish hebephrenic from paranoid patients. He concludes that 'the distinctive behaviour of each of these sub-types appears to be a different way of responding to the same basic difficulty' (Shakow, 1962). He suggests that the clinical phenomena represent different forms of reaction to the psychological disorganization which characterizes schizophrenic patients. In the hebephrenic patient there is no effort to deal with this deterioration, whereas in the paranoid case the response takes the form of an over-reaction against the disorganization of mental life.

This theory is very close to Freud's view that the well-formed delusional ideation characteristic of the paranoid schizophrenic is in the nature of a restitutional process whereby the patient attempts to re-order and re-organize his cognition so that it can accommodate the alterations made by the psychosis in his means of representing his conception of self and the object world (see Chapter 2). Freud (1924) put this theory in another way when he said that the delusion is ' . . . like a patch on the spot where originally there was a rent in the relation between ego and outer world'. This enables the patient to continue in some kind of adaptation to the environment. Hebephrenic illnesses are without adequate restitutional methods.

The work of Shakow (1962) and other experimentalists has also revealed data which accord with those reported by many psychoanalytical investigators. A patient who suffers from a psychosis exhibits a symptom and behavioural complex which cannot be equated with the symptoms and signs of the vast majority of physical diseases. Whereas the former are characterized by a fluidity and variation in the symptomatology, the latter are invariably constant and unchanging both within the one patient and from patient to patient. There is, in Shakow's (1962) words, little inter- or intra-patient variability. Psycho-analysis predicted such variability in its theory that there is a constant process of regression and disorganization occurring *pari passu* with a restitutional trend. Psychological research in the psychoses cannot afford to ignore this phenomenological variability. Psycho-analytic theory alerts the investigator to its presence and possible causes.

Psycho-analysis has been frequently criticized for its indifferent attitude to the formal characteristics of clinical phenomena. It is sometimes said that psycho-analysts have no interest in symptoms. Today psychopathology is often regarded as synonymous with psychoanalytical formulations of unconscious phantasy and conflict. This is incorrect, and psycho-analysts would suggest that this view has arisen from a one-sided understanding of psycho-analysis. Initially, primary emphasis was laid in psycho-analysis on unconscious mental contents because of their relationship to symptoms (the dynamic factor), but this was soon complemented by attempts to understand those other factors which were responsible for the form which mental processes assume. Freud's metapsychological theory (1915) was an attempt to accommodate all aspects of mental functioning. Psychopathology began as the study of the experiences which patients reported as symptoms, while most psycho-analytical formulations are in the nature of inferences which have been abstracted from the clinical phenomena. They are thus data of a qualitatively different order from the symptoms themselves.

Psycho-analysis is by no means indifferent to symptoms and other contents of consciousness. Readers of *The Interpretation of Dreams* (Freud, 1900) will note that the analysis of a dream begins from the manifest content, and this only with the co-operation of the dreamer. In this work Freud was concerned with examining the particular form which the dream images assumed. He stated (1900) ' . . . if we wish to pursue our study of the relations between dream content and dream thoughts further, the best plan will be to take dreams themselves as our point of departure and consider what certain formal characteristics of the method of representation in dreams signify in relation to the thoughts underlying them. Most prominent among the formal characteristics, which cannot fail to impress us in dreams, are the differences in sensory intensity between particular dream images and in the distinctness of particular parts of dreams or whole dreams as compared with one another.' This quotation illustrates a characteristic found throughout Freud's writings of commencing with an examination of the manifest phenomena and then proceeding to the construction of hypotheses regarding the means of their formation.

A psycho-analytical approach to the psychoses can be rewarding in clinical and research studies if full use is made of the theoretical concepts which Freud elaborated in *The Interpretation of Dreams* and in articles published between 1911 and 1916. The objection may be raised that this approach puts 'the cart before the horse' — the theoretical constructs influencing the selection of the phenomena which are necessary to give them validity. Even allowing for this objection, there remains the fact that without hypothesis clinical observations remain disconnected and meaningless. With the help of a theoretical model isolated groups of data can be converted into a series which bear a consistent relationship to one another. This relationship need not be a causal one. It is not the adoption of a model that makes for difficulties, but the possibility that the investigator's preference for a particular conceptual system will unconsciously influence him in the selection of material. On the other hand, difficulty in accepting a hypothesis and the need to find data to discredit it can spring from unconscious sources within the observer. In the last resort it will be the integrity of the observer which will decide whether or not a hypothetical construct proves to be a liability or an asset. When confronted with phenomena which run counter to theoretical expectations he must be prepared to re-examine his hypotheses.

Psycho-analysis impinges upon a number of other disciplines. Psycho-analysis and genetic psychology are at one in their emphasis upon the developmental aspects of mental function, with all the implications this has for primitivization and disorganization. At this point there is contiguity with the dissolution-evolution hypothesis of nervous system activity. It is now known (Jones, 1953) that Freud leant heavily on this theory of Hughlings Jackson in the elaboration of his concept of regression and his other developmental hypotheses. By virtue of its instinct theory, psycho-analysis, as Stengel (1954) has pointed out, has not been confined to a purely psychogenic aetiology of the neuroses and psychoses. Again, the biological base of psycho-analysis has been re-affirmed by Bowlby (1960), Szekely (1954), and others who have studied the behaviour of infants and young children using the concepts of psycho-analysis and ethology.

Freud's concepts were designed to present as comprehensive a view as possible of the manner in which mental processes operate. However, his discovery of the dynamic nature of mental life was so revolutionary that for long enough priority has been afforded to this aspect of mental activity in psycho-analytic theorizing. Conflict, repression, and the impact of the repressed upon the contents of consciousness are concepts which until recently have dominated the psycho-analytical scene. While these concepts are invaluable for the understanding and treatment of the psychoneuroses, they cannot be given priority in psychotic states. Concepts that are essential in the neuroses are insufficient to describe the process at work in psychotic reactions. The dynamic interpretation of a psychotic symptom, emphasizing, as it does, the influence of the repressed, needs to be supplemented by an account of the other non-dynamic processes which Freud conceptualized as structural, economic, and topographical respectively.

The understanding of Freud's metapsychology has been simplified by Rapaport's (1951) elucidation of the concepts which comprise this theory. In the process of this clarification he has laid emphasis on Freud's insistence on not giving priority to mental content in assessing the relative importance of the factors which lead to psychological phenomena. In a footnote to *The Interpretation of Dreams*, Freud stated (1955) ' . . . now that analysts at least have become reconciled to replacing the manifest dream by the meaning revealed by its interpretation, many of them have become guilty of falling into another confusion which they cling to with equal obstinacy. They seek to find the essence of dreams in their latent content, and in so doing they overlook the distinction between the latent dream thoughts and the dream work. At bottom, dreams are nothing other than a particular form of thinking, made possible by the conditions of the state of sleep. It is the dream work which creates that form, and it alone is the essence of dreaming – the explanation of its peculiar nature.' In this quotation Freud relegates content (latent dream content) to a secondary place in favour of the mental processes which undertake the dream work.

The lack of interest in the form and operation of mental processes has been offset during the past twenty years by the development of psycho-analytic ego psychology. Hartmann (1939) initiated this interest with his monograph *Ego Psychology and the Problem of Adaptation*. The basic ideas for this ego psychology originated in observations made by Freud in one of his last papers. In this article, Freud (1937) departed from his earlier views by stressing an entirely different aspect of ego development. This 'new look' was not incompatible with his earlier conceptions but rather complemented the latter in a manner which was to facilitate the bridging of the gap between psycho-analysis and general psychology. Briefly, Freud proposed that the form and functioning of the ego in maturity will be dependent on hereditary influences. The traits which characterize the adult ego – and this refers to preference in defence mechanisms, to the form of perceptual and thought processes – are determined by two factors. First, the hereditary factor and second, the defensive conflicts which are necessary if the individual is to achieve a *modus vivendi* with his instinctual aims on the one hand and the environment on the other. As Freud (1937) puts it

B

' . . . we recognize that the peculiarities of the ego which we detect in the form of resistances may be not only acquired in defence conflicts but (also) determined by heredity . . . '

Hartmann (1939) proposed that ego functions – the secondary process of Freud's (1900) original terminology – have autonomous roots independent of conflict. These sources are outside the sphere of conflict – described by Hartmann as ' . . . the conflict-free ego sphere'. The maturation of these ego functions is dependent on laws which are part of the individual's inheritance. This concept of autonomous ego functions is one which has lessened the distance between psycho-analysis and general psychology. It has reduced some of the difficulty which non-analytical psychologists have had in their understanding of psycho-analysis. This has arisen because of doubts about accepting a theory of mental function which seemed to regard every cognitive function and every personality trait as originating in conflict. Hartmann's theory had an earlier counterpart in Schilder's (1923) assertion that all mental functions – particularly cognition – could not be traced to drive derivatives and to the conflicts to which they give rise. This is clear in the following quotation: 'Though we treat thinking under the heading of drive theory we must be aware that there are structures related to thinking which cannot be explained by genetic constructions. The very existence of images, thoughts, judgements is in point. Moreover though affects and drives do play a most significant role even in perception, there are aspects of perception which are totally independent of any drive' (Schilder, 1923).

The advent of the ego-autonomy concept has led to a renewed interest in cognitive (ego) functioning and this is reflected in a number of clinical and experimental studies conducted by psycho-analytically trained psychologists. Work of this type is particularly relevant for the problem of psychosis, since it is in these states that cognition may be seriously deranged. The best known of these applied psycho-analytic researches are those of Klein (1954), Gardiner (1962), and Holzman (1954). The effect of this work has been to redirect attention to Freud's original views about the role of consciousness and to the factors which determine its functional states. An indispensable feature of these hypotheses is the consideration given to the non-dynamic aspects of mental processes.

Klein (1959) has this to say ' . . . there are processes other than repression (in the sense of a pushing out) which deny them (that is the mental representations of sensory stimuli) awareness or attention cathexis. But what is the relationship of such non-conscious events to repression in the usual sense? Psycho-analytical theory has tended to emphasize repressed contents and has ignored the wider array of non-experienced contents which may be simply the outcome of the workings of perception and other presentational modes in different states of consciousness, rather than of repression.' This conclusion has important relevances for such schizophrenic manifestations as distractability, lack of attentive capacity, and faulty concentration.

The results of the experimental work referred to suggest that, with visual perception at least, a series of non-conscious events take place prior to the emergence of a percept or image in consciousness. Fisher (1956) has shown that the memory trace of a visual stimulus may be subjected to transformations and to other alterations. He has pointed out that these changes are the result of the impact of the primary process. In the pre-stages of visual perception the dominating influences are condensation and displacement. Referring to developmental aspects of perceptual and memory functions Fisher says ' . . . there are early phases during which they are capable of functioning only in certain ways, for example with condensation and displacements. These early mechanisms do not disappear with further development, but are simply overlaid by more mature reality oriented perceptual and memory processes. Furthermore these early phases persist in the organism and constitute preliminary stages in the development of reality orientated percepts and memories.' It would appear that there is no conscious mental activity which does not have an unconscious development. This was Freud's (1900) original position as evidenced by his statement ' . . . everything conscious has an unconscious preliminary stage . . . ' This must apply as much to external perception as to the awareness of the mental representation of the drives.

A further consequence of Hartmann's work has been that psychoanalysts have become interested in the work of psychologists who have studied the development of cognitive functions. Piaget's (1947) account of sensorimotor development in the early months of life appears to supplement current psycho-analytical views on the growth of the ego functions in the first year of life. His concept of sensori-motor schemata provides a means of describing the observable phenomena in a meaningful way. The development of the schema of the permanent object can be usefully compared with psycho-analytical hypotheses regarding the beginnings of object relationships. The schema of the object does not achieve effective functioning until the eighth month of life. It is at this time, according to psycho-analytical observers, that it is no longer possible to substitute nurse for mother, or mother for nurse, without distressing the infant. Piaget's observations also provide support for Hartmann's assertion that perceptual and motor activities arise independently of the infant's needs and that they are only secondarily put at the service of these needs.

Piaget's concept of assimilation and accommodation can also be likened to the psycho-analytic concepts of introjection and projection. Assimilation describes an infantile mode of mental functioning whereby the individual registers all manner of environmental impressions. In this way there is an expansion of the developing personality. At a later stage the mechanism of accommodation operates to structure the incoming data, to isolate and delete what is irrelevant for environmental adaptation. Introjection describes the same process as assimilation, and projection has some of the characteristics of accommodation. Accommodation implies the operation of threshold mechanisms (inhibition in neurophysiology (Lindsley, 1960) – countercathexes (Rapaport, 1951) in psycho-analytic theory) which limit the intrusion into consciousness of data that would interfere with relevant responses and directed thinking. These concepts are important for a psychological theory of schizophrenia because many patients appear to have lost the capacity to restrict the influx of external and internal stimuli.

Today psycho-analysis takes full cognizance of the developments which are taking place in experimental and genetic psychology, the more so because many of the findings and concepts are in line with the basic theories of psycho-analysis. The work of experimental and genetic psychologists provides information about the form which mental processes assume, how these forms alter during the course of development, and how they are influenced by the impact of extraneous and internal stimulation. Such data must be available to the psycho-analytic investigator because in the psychoses it is the formal aspect of mental activity – particularly of cognition – which is disturbed.

Psycho-analysts must acquaint themselves with the data and concepts of psychology and psychophysiology if they are to make a serious contribution to research in the psychoses. In its practical aspects psycho-analysis is a clinical method, and it is this which imposes a serious limitation upon its capacity to solve the psychosis problem by itself. The failure of the clinical method in psychiatry to make a fundamental contribution to nosology and aetiology arises from the nature of the subject-matter. The psychotic patient does not recognize the significance of his abnormal experiences and sees no reason why he should talk about them. In this respect he is quite unlike the patient who suffers from a physical ailment. In cases of schizophrenia, data of decisive significance for the isolation of syndromes either do not appear at all or appear only after a very long period of contact between patient and physician. Another difficulty arises from the fact that interpretation of these data often varies from one experienced clinician to another. Everyone agrees on the necessity of employing test procedures and continually trying to construct psychological and psychophysiological methods that will lead to the exposure of data capable of becoming as diagnostically significant as the volume and diameter of the red blood-cell in a case of anaemia. Thus far the examination of tests has been confined to groups of patients and the results compared with healthy controls. This research has not fulfilled its promise as far as the individual patient is concerned.

One chapter (Chapter 9) of this book is devoted to an account of the psychological approach that has been employed in the study of schizophrenic patients. These methods were devised in the hope that they would provide information not available in the clinical setting and that they would be less subject to observer error than is the clinical method. Recognition of the need for assistance from other disciplines in no way diminishes the extent of the psycho-analytic contribution. This rests essentially on the demonstration of the background of the individual patient's subjective responses and his reactions to experimental situations. It was the psycho-analyst who was the first to see that much current psychological research suffers from its decision to ignore, however temporarily, what Shakow (1962) has referred to as the 'attitude' variable. It is claimed that this decision has arisen from the difficulty of elucidating the endopsychic factors that constitute the 'attitude' variable and designing experiments which can bring them under control. While this is a real difficulty, it merely underlines the need for further detailed descriptive and psycho-analytic studies of individual patients' reactions to test situations (see Chapter 7).

Psychiatric knowledge is still at a stage when exploratory research is vitally important and phenomenological studies must be pursued with vigour. It is only through such studies that recurring complexes of phenomena can be identified. The results of these inquiries may help towards the construction of experiments designed to make manifest the operation of the factors that constitute the 'attitude' variable and influence a patient in his test performance. Fruitful results in psychosis research will come about only when the clinical and experimental methods are jointly utilized. Each approach acts as a corrective to the other and at the same time supplements what is lacking in the other discipline.

CHAPTER 2

Psycho-analytic Theories of Psychosis

Psycho-analytic theories of psychosis consist essentially of the idea that the patient's mental activity operates at different functional levels. It is the confluence of disorganized adult mental processes, on the one hand, with undifferentiated syncretic processes, on the other, that leads to the patient's failure to maintain environmental adaptation. The concepts on which the theories are based are designed to identify phenomena arising from the various 'developmental' layers. The conceptual scheme advanced by psycho-analysis with respect to the psychoses goes a great deal further in facilitating the description of clinical data than is possible with a framework which regards the clinical data as due entirely to the outcome of a disorganization of adult mental activity.

THE CLASSICAL THEORY

The essential features of the theory described by Freud (1911) consist, first, of a disruption of the patient's relationship with the world of objects and, second, of an attempt to re-organize and re-structure this defective relationship capacity. Freud couched his hypothesis in terms of the libido theory which he had formulated for the neuroses. This theory of psychosis (1911) antedated his structural concepts of ego, id, and superego by about twelve years. This is important, because the use of the term ego in 1911 was different from his conception of the ego later described in *The Ego and the Id* (1923). The ego concept (1923) is central for current psycho-analytic theories of psychosis.

In this first systematic presentation of a psycho-analytic theory of psychosis, Freud (1911) was principally concerned with the illness described then as paranoia and with giving an explanation of the contents of the persecutory delusions. Indeed, the details now known about Schreber's illness would incline most psychiatrists to consider his condition as one of paranoid schizophrenia. Freud (1911) elaborated upon hypothesized mechanisms which governed the onset and development of paranoia. In order to do this, he conceived of a process comparable to repression in which libidinal cathexes were withdrawn from the world of objects and their intrapsychic representations. This withdrawal and detachment of cathexes did not have to be complete — it could be partial — the patient retaining some capacity for object cathexis.

This comparison with repression was appropriate because repression in the healthy and in the psychoneurotic individual is conceived of as a withdrawal of cathexes from preconscious verbal representations. Freud was merely extending this concept to the field of the psychoses. The process that commenced with the withdrawal of cathexes from objects was followed by a regression, in cases of paranoia, to a narcissistic state. By this time the second phase was already in operation — the process of restitution, to use Freud's terminology.

The restitutional phase was envisaged as consisting of an attempt to regain the lost object world. The special contents of this phase suggested that it could be compared with the psychoneuroses, where, with the failure of repression, there is a return, in a distorted and unrecognized form, of what had previously been repressed. Freud (1911) suggested that the mechanism of projection was the means whereby the restitutional process operated in cases of paranoia. He understood the schizophrenias as being due to an even greater cathectic disturbance and to a regression to an objectless auto-erotic phase. Restitution in such cases depended upon hallucinatory mechanisms rather than upon projection. The projection mechanism enabled the patient to externalize wishes which were unacceptable to him. It thus provided the conditions for the content of the persecutory delusions. Freud proposed that the hallucinatory experiences which the schizophrenic patient complained of were in fact revived memory traces now experienced as auditory or visual percepts.

The prototype of this mechanism was the theory of hallucinatory wish-fulfilment envisaged as occurring in the infant who is impatient for food. The wish for food stimulates memory traces of past satisfactions and brings them to hallucinatory vividness. Freud (1900) described this mechanism of hallucination as a form of topographic regression. The drive energy (cathexis) was directed to the sensory (perceptual) end of the mental apparatus rather than to the motor system. The concept of topographic regression was employed by Freud (1900) to account for the visual images of the dream. In schizophrenia the patient tried to restore his lost object relations by substituting the memory of objects in hallucinatory form which were both real and phantasy, pleasurable and distressing. Those cases who showed both delusions and hallucinations employed both projection and topographic regression as restitutional measures.

In a later paper (1915) Freud proposed that the disturbance of conceptual thinking in schizophrenia was likewise due to a withdrawal of cathexes from endopsychic object representation. As a measure of restitution the cathexes were directed to the memory traces of words which were no longer tied to their appropriate object. The verbal symbol no longer represented its appropriate object. Words were now cathected and treated concretely by the patient, and used without regard to their correct significance. Freud discussed the thinking disorder in psychosis again in 1916, when he stated that topographic regression does not occur in schizophrenia. In dreams there is free communication of cathexes between the mental representation of objects and their appropriate verbal symbols, whereas in the schizo-prenias this communication is broken off. In schizophrenia the word representations (the verbal symbols) are subject to the primary process and not the mental representation of objects as in dreams.

A close reading of Freud's paper suggests that his statement that topographic regression does not occur in schizophrenia refers only to the change which has taken place in the thought processes in schizo-phrenia and not to the hallucinatory phenomena. Clinical reports show the frequency with which images and memory traces are revived as hallucinations in psychoses (see Chapter 6). This suggests, as men-tioned above, that in hallucinatory states a topographic regression to the perceptual apparatus occurs along similar lines to that of the dream. Freud (1916) states ' . . . we may be allowed to assume that hallucina-tions consist in a cathexis of the system Conscious (Pcpt) which however does not proceed — as normally — from without but from within, the condition being that regression shall be carried far enough to reach this system itself and thus to pass beyond the testing of reality'.

In the same paper (1916) Freud has further comments to make upon the role played by regression in the formation of clinical hallucinations. His remarks have a greater importance because they take up the ques-tion of reality-testing, the failure of which leads to hallucination and delusion. In the dream the regressive movement of cathexis innervates the perceptual apparatus and leads to the pictorial presentation of memory traces. In waking life the regressive revival of memory images does not lead to hallucination. This is due to the function of reality-testing, which differentiates images from percepts. As Freud (1916) points out, 'This capacity did not always exist and that at the beginning of our mental life we really hallucinated the satisfying object when we felt the need of it. But even so, satisfaction remained lacking and this failure must have moved us to create some faculty to help us to distinguish such a wish perception from an actual fulfilment and to avoid it for the future. In other words we gave up hallucinatory gratification of our wishes at a very early period and established a kind of testing of reality.' It may be said, therefore, that the testing of reality is in some way bound up with the capacity to discriminate between ideational activity on the one hand and perceptual experience on the other.

Today psycho-analytic theoreticians no longer regard object cath-exes as being principally composed of libidinal energies. Following upon Freud's later instinct theory, which postulated destructive and libidinal drives, Hartmann (1952) and others proposed that the object cathexes which 'energize' object relations in the healthy have been subject to neutralization. They have been 'de-instinctualized'. During development, instinctual forces are subjected to a process of neutraliza-tion—this particularly applies to the aggressive drives, the neutralization of which provides the energy that activates the ego and its function of environmental adaptation. In pathological states the drives may become de-neutralized and regain their instinctual quality.This excursion into the realms of psycho-analytical theory is not as academic as might at first appear, because it is no longer possible to conceive object relation-ships in the mentally ill or in the healthy as being entirely driven by libidinal energy. The clinical fact is that conflicts regarding destructive tendencies occupy a large part of the patient's preoccupations and symptomatology.

This concern with the nature of object cathexes has another impor-tant facet, which is closely linked with the concept of narcissism, which plays such an important part in psycho-analytic theories of psychosis. It is necessary, therefore, to give some initial consideration to this con-cept not only in its pathological forms but also in its developmental aspects. Narcissism is inseparably connected with the sense of self and awareness of self. Clinical psycho-analysis has shown that pathological narcissism — an exaggerated evaluation of the self — arises on the basis of disturbed object relationships in early childhood. Failure to obtain suitable objects that can become the recipients of object cathexes results in a tendency towards concentrating these cathexes upon the developing self. This process has essentially a defensive function because the enhanced self-love protects against disappointment with objects. A further disadvantageous consequence occurring simultaneously, and facilitated by the pathological narcissism, is the trend to replace an active object-seeking drive by passivity in object relationships. Passivity is an important characteristic of pathological narcissism. Under normal conditions narcissism — love of self — is controlled by the development of object relations. In Freud's (1914) original formulation narcissistic libido is converted into object libido. A certain quantity of narcissism is left which ensures self-esteem and pleasure in self.

For those who are characterized by a powerful narcissism as a consequence of disturbed and disordered childhood relations, the choice of object in later life tends to be made on a narcissistic basis. That is to say that the model for the chosen object is the conception of the self — either actual or wished for. It follows that all the relationships of a narcissistically orientated individual will reflect aspects of the self — all objects will be appendages of the self and treated as such. This means that others cannot be treated as individuals in their own right because these others are not invested with object libidinal cathexes but with narcissistic cathexes. A few psycho-analytical writers since Freud, perhaps Federn (1953) is the outstanding example, have pointed out that object cathexes, which optimally should be composed of a mixture of instinctual (libidinal) and neutralized libidinal and aggressive energies will, in the narcissistically fixated individual, be composed of narcissistic (instinctual-libidinal) cathexes. This hypothesis has an important implication for psycho-analytic theories of psychosis.

Earlier a reference was made to that aspect of psycho-analytic theory which proposes that in the psychoses there is a regression to a narcissistic state. Controversy among psycho-analysts centres upon the question of the nature and the function of this narcissism. The question is, how does this psychotic narcissism relate to normal narcissism, to the narcissism of the sexually deviant, and to the narcissism of those whose personalities are severely disturbed? There is clinical evidence to suggest that a similarity exists between the narcissism of the psychotic patient in the pre-psychotic phase and the other narcissistic states. Whether this identity continues with the onset of the psychosis is another matter. It may be that the narcissism of the established psychotic state, to which Freud refers in his original hypothesis, is something quite different from that encountered in the sexual deviations and the character abnormalities. Katan (1954), as is well known, has described what he calls a narcissistic form of the oedipus complex where the heterosexual object is endowed with the patient's femininity.

Narcissism was described by Freud on one occasion as the libidinal component of egoism. This statement emphasizes the egocentrism which is an inherent feature of the concept. This egocentrism is most apparent in the psychotic patient and it constitutes the core of the series of phenomena that characterize this pathological state. Details of these data will be given later. This pathological egocentrism has much in common with the egocentrism of the young child who cannot conceive of events as occurring outside a relationship to himself.

At the present time a psycho-analytic theory of psychosis is dependent upon the structural concepts introduced by Freud in 1923 — particularly the concepts of ego and superego. The majority of psychoanalytical writers on the psychoses refer to these conditions as mental states which can be explained on the basis of a serious ego disintegration affecting the processes serving environmental adaptation and defence against the instinctual drives. It is worth recalling that this interest in ego dysfunction in psychoses was pioneered by Federn (1943), who thought that an ego insufficiency — deficiency of ego cathexes — was the principal factor leading to the psychotic symptomatology.

It is perhaps appropriate here to refer to an important amendment which Federn (1943) made to Freud's original theory of psychosis. According to Freud (1911), the withdrawal and detachment of object (narcissistic) cathexes was the first — 'silent' — step on the path to symptom formation. Distorted perception of self and the world followed the regression, which affected the ego. Federn (1948) disagreed with this view. He felt that the withdrawal from the object world was a consequence of the ego defect and not the cause of it. He presented clinical data which showed that patients at the onset of the illness falsified and distorted perceptual experiences while still having a relationship with objects. This observation can easily be confirmed in patients who will interpret a lapse of memory as due to interference from without rather than recognize the true cause — an unconscious wish not to remember.

In Federn's (1943) opinion, these disturbances of perceptual experience can often be traced to some special incident antedating the distortion by minutes or hours. A knowledge of the background to such occurrences can sometimes be turned to therapeutic advantage. In the example quoted, the memory lapse may be explored and the patient's unconscious tendency to deal with painful affects by repression and subsequent projection brought to light. In such a case the patient may retain the capacity to relate, and this enables the successful analysis of the symptom to be undertaken.

The disagreement between the two views is more apparent than real, because Freud's theory (1911) proposed that there was not a complete detachment and withdrawal of cathexes from objects. The withdrawal of cathexes occurred simultaneously with the disorganization within the ego. This theory can therefore explain the simultaneous falsification of perceptual experience due to ego defect while object relations are still partially retained. The ego concept which Freud introduced in 1923 was necessary in view of the phenomenon of unconscious resistance. Resistance arose from the ego, and yet this was unconscious. Consciousness and ego could no longer be equated, nor could the system Unconscious of the topographic terminology be regarded as completely lacking differentiation if functions of the ego arose from it. The superego concept facilitated the integration of the idea of an unconscious conscience, and received support from clinical observation. Apart from these considerations, the ego concept enabled Freud (1923) to define what he regarded as the essence of the ego — its functions in the adult and how it came into being.

PSYCHOSIS AS THE RESULT OF EGO DEFECT

In contrast to the earlier usage, Freud described the ego in 1923 as 'a coherent organisation of mental processes'. The ego processes were to be distinguished from the processes of the id (system Unconscious), which were undifferentiated and unorganized. Werner's (1948) concept of syncretism, which stresses the lack of differentiation between mental processes, describes the state of unconscious mentation. It can be equated with the mechanisms of the primary process — condensation and displacement. The ego functions comprise those mental activities which are usually grouped together and described as cognition. Thinking, perceiving, remembering, insight, judgement, attending, concentrating, sense of self, and awareness of self are all ego functions. To these must be added the mechanisms of defence.

For some time after the introduction of the ego concept it was thought that ego functions developed as a consequence of the identifications that followed upon close interpersonal relationships. Freud (1923) described the ego on one occasion as the precipitate of past object choices. This formulation provides an explanation of character traits and personality attitudes. The ego was thought to develop out of conflict – when the object had to be renounced it was internalized in the ego. In recent years, as was mentioned in the introductory chapter, a new theory has arisen which helps to explain the development of cognition in contrast to personality characteristics.

The theory of autonomous ego development has brought psychoanalysis into close contact with the genetic psychologies of Werner and Piaget, who both look upon adult cognition as being the end-product of a developmental process beginning at a sensori-motor level and ending at a conceptual level. In infancy mental processes – thinking, perceiving, motor activity – are not differentiated. There is no inhibitory influence preventing the spread of a stimulus from the perceptual to the motor apparatus. This inhibition develops gradually and is the mechanism which Freud described as characteristic of the secondary process. Sensory experience is likewise characterized by lack of discrimination between the different sensory modalities. Hearing, seeing, and sensations of all kinds are not differentiated, hence the phenomenon of synaesthesia frequently observed in children and even in adults under special conditions. Differentiation of the various sensory modalities occurs with growth, as does the development of size and object constancy in the sphere of visual perception.

Perception of sensation and external impressions which mirror internal and external conditions is primarily dependent upon the growth of self as a discrete entity distinct from other environmental entities. Piaget (1932) has described this infantile state as one of adualism. The child does not discriminate between the self and objects. Freud in his 'primary identification', postulated a similar concept to that of Piaget. According to this the first object relationships of the child are not distinguished from the self but are part of it. There is no clear distinction between external and internal with regard to the perception of sensations. Federn (1953) described this discriminating function as that of the ego boundary – a term borrowed from Tausk (1919), who used it in the description and interpretation of a case of schizophrenia.

In its earliest phases, therefore, the ego is not characterized by discriminatory capacities of a high order. Sense of self and recognition of self as an entity are rudimentary. At this point the instinctual and structural aspects of the theory of mental development meet, because in the young infant the absence of established ego boundaries (primary identification) is contemporaneous with a fleeting sense of self which is, nevertheless, the centre of all experience. This has been described as the period of primary narcissism, to distinguish it from the later secondary narcissism which appears with the growth of object relations after self-object discrimination has been established.

Further elaboration of the ego function of self-awareness and sense of identity was made by Federn (1949) and in more recent times by Jacobson (1954). Federn (1949) thought that the sense of identity and what he described as 'ego feeling' were dependent upon an adequate cathexis of the ego and of its boundaries. Loss of the ego-boundary cathexis led to the absence of sensation and feeling which characterizes the phenomena of depersonalization, while a deficiency of the ego cathexis led to the symptoms of psychosis.

Jacobson (1954a) introduced the concept of self-representation to complement the concept of object-representations. The growth of self-representations is dependent upon the type and form of object relationships which occur in infancy and childhood. Adequate self-representations will depend upon a sound discrimination between self and object and upon the limitation of primary narcissism. This, as has been pointed out, can occur only when there is the opportunity for the instinctual drives to invest objects in infancy with cathexis. The concept of self-representations is therefore closely linked with those of narcissism, primary identification, and the ego boundary. It also has close associations with perception of the body, in contrast to the awareness of mental experience. Federn's (1948) hypothesis of mental and bodily ego feeling are particularly useful, making as they do this important distinction.

Awareness of self, the capacity to reflect upon one's experiences, is dependent upon an intact ego. This capacity is weakened in dreams, although it is not extinguished. It is also altered in anaesthesia, anoxaemia, and similar conditions. A realistic appraisal of the environment is dependent upon adequate reflective awareness. Concentration and attention, which are necessary to bring this about, demand that ego functions remain intact. The state of consciousness correlates with the condition of self-awareness. As self-awareness diminishes, the state of consciousness alters and is no longer adequate for the task of purposive attention and concentration. Coincidental with the loss of self-awareness is the disappearance of the discriminating function between self and object (ego boundaries). Similarly, experience of the body also changes with damage to the ego. The body schema is yet another ego function which develops contemporaneously with the increasing discriminatory and inhibitory tendencies that characterize the developing ego. Injury to the ego leads to loss of inhibition and to failure of discrimination.

During the earliest phases of ego development, thinking, although having autonomous origins, becomes linked with the instinctual needs. Memory traces of satisfactory and pleasurable experiences become cathected whenever the infant is in a state of need. Initially, it is hypothesized, these memory traces are experienced as percepts (hallucinatory gratification). For a long time ideation is tied to the drives and can be described as 'drive orientated' to use Rapaport's (1951) expression. Environmental objects, whether animate or inanimate, come to have powerful affective and instinctual associations which may give rise to either pleasure or anxiety. The capacity to utilize verbal symbols for communication depends upon these symbols not only representing specific objects but also becoming separated off from the earlier affect and drive associations of the objects they have come to signify.

During ego development, thinking passes from a sensori-motor level to a perceptual and finally to a conceptual level (Werner, 1948). At the sensori-motor level, thought processes are 'instinct driven' and are concerned only with need satisfaction and the avoidance of excessive sensory stimulation. At the perceptual level, thinking is tied to the immediate situation in which the child finds himself and is therefore essentially concrete. In the conceptual phase, verbal symbols allow the child to detach himself from perceptual stimuli. Thinking is now autonomous and a high degree of abstraction is possible. In the sensori-motor phase, thought processes are a facet of the sensori-motor activity which is the behavioural mode. Thinking, like perceiving, passes through developmental stages which are governed by an increasing discrimination and inhibition. According to psycho-analytic theory, conceptual thinking is energized by neutralized drive cathexis, in contrast to earlier forms of mentation, which are activated by instinctual energies governed by the laws of the primary process.

Over the years, psychiatrists and psycho-analysts have observed phenomena in cases of psychosis which can be interpreted as a revival of mental activity appropriate to earlier phases of ego development. No claim has been made for a complete identity between the clinical data and the developmental phenomena encountered in the healthy child. Each shows a striking similarity to the other, and it is thus reasonable to assume that the phenomena which appear in the psychotic state are partly due to a regression affecting ego functions. These phenomena may arise in any of the ego activities to which reference has been made.

The disturbances may consist of a loss of self-object discrimination or of a loss of the autonomy and independence of the self. The sense of identity may be impaired and replaced by a mixture of self- and object-representations. Faulty discrimination may lead to states of consciousness characterized by a massive assimilation of environmental stimuli which then constitute the content of the patient's communications. This is akin to the childhood state where fragments of overheard speech are incorporated into verbal utterances. Distractability also arises from the inability to screen out excessive external stimulation.

In the sphere of thinking, forms analogous to those of early developmental phases appear, especially in cases of hebephrenic schizophrenia. The capacity to form concepts is often seriously disturbed. Abstract ideas, objects, and events are no longer adequately discriminated by their verbal symbols. The symbols themselves, as a result of condensation, acquire different meanings. Thinking in these instances has now assumed the earlier dependence upon the drives for its activation. Words frequently become concretized and are regarded by the patient as objects. This is, however, not as common a phenomenon as is sometimes claimed. A tendency to concrete thinking, which is so common in childhood is, as is probably true of the schizophrenic patient also, the outcome of the perceptual level at which thinking operates.

In the motor-perceptual sphere, many patients demonstrate a loss of the inhibitory forces which separate stimulus from response. Just as the child responds to perceptual stimulation with bodily responses and not with verbal communication, so do many schizophrenic patients react to verbal stimuli with bodily movements. Echopraxia belongs to this category of phenomena. No limitation is imposed upon the response to the visual percept of the other person's movement. These impressions are assimilated indiscriminately, owing to the deficiencies in the boundary functions of the ego, which should perform the task of excluding stimuli that may lead to non-adaptive thought and behaviour. Once assimilated, the percepts lead to immediate motor responses – the echopractic movement.

The sensory modalities may be so affected that vision and hearing are not discriminated by the patient. Identical motor responses may

C

arise from either stimulus. The patient may state that his reaction to a visual percept is identical with that to an auditory stimulus. This phenomenon has been termed 'functional equivalence' by the genetic psychologists. Equally striking are those patients who find that genital sensations are confused with tactile, auditory, or visual stimuli. These stimuli may be actual or hallucinatory in nature. These phenomena have close associations with childhood phases of development and with the experience of some healthy adults. The same can be said for aspects of schizophrenic thinking, because even in the mentally healthy there is a tendency to corrupt verbal expression, to concretize, and to utilize primary process mechanisms as, for example, in humour and colloquialism. It is most important, as Bleuler (1963) has recently pointed out, to be constantly aware of the common ground which exists between the schizophrenic patient and the mentally normal adult. Again, it is not uncommon for the hebephrenic patient to report disturbances of size and shape constancy. Faces, bodies, objects become bigger, smaller, or change in shape.

All the phenomena to which reference has been made can be legitimately regarded as products of regression following ego injury. An exception of this generalization is to be found in the neurological signs that may be detected in patients who are usually diagnosed as hebephrenic or catatonic schizophrenias. When the illness is well established these patients show, as Schilder (1928) demonstrated many years ago, a disorganization of neurological function which bears no similarity to any developmental phase of normal childhood. In such cases it is not uncommon to discover the presence of the 'catatonic pupil' which fails to constrict in response to a light stimulus. The flexor muscles are often characterized by a hypertonicity and the tendon reflexes strikingly accentuated. A gross inequality of reflex response between right and left sides is occasionally encountered and this reflex activity is influenced by posture. It is also possible to demonstrate sensory impairments (sensory inattention).

These phenomena cannot be attributed entirely to the effects of protracted hospitalization, as has often been done. These signs appear even when the patient is given a great deal of attention and the hospitalization effect is reduced to a minimum. In cases demonstrating these signs, the neurological disorganization is matched in its extent by the disorganization that affects every sphere of psychological functioning. It seems unlikely that these neurological manifestations can be considered as the products of regression.

RECENT THEORIES

The assumption made by some psycho-analysts (see below) that all schizophrenic phenomena are regressive in nature entails the view that they are not 'end products' but only the surface expression of hidden conflicts in the sphere of object relations, in much the same manner as psychoneurotic symptoms are the substitute for unconscious conflicts. There is general agreement among psycho-analysts on two points. First, that the patient's disturbed cognition or delusional ideas represent a communication and, second, that the analyst-patient situation can become the focus for the concentration of conflicts arising out of object-relationship difficulties. In this way the latter can be studied in their association with symptomatological changes. As this discussion relates at this point to the functional level of cognition, no reference will be made now to those reports which deal with delusions and with altera-tions in their content.

The purpose of numerous psycho-analytic publications (Rosenfeld, 1952; Bion, 1957, 1959; Searles, 1959a) has been to demonstrate two things. First, how a cognitive upset can be regarded as a reflection of, and a response to, a particular form of object relationship and, second, how an alteration in the quality of an object relationship can lead to changes in a specific cognitive function. In every case the clinical phenomena appear within the context of the patient-analyst situation. They are, in these reports, regarded as manifestations of transferences (transference psychosis) from the earliest infantile period. It is important to examine these conceptualizations, because they are hypotheses designed to explain the mechanism of schizophrenic symptomatology.

All psycho-analytical theories of schizophrenia regard the regressive process as primarily a defence against anxiety and guilt activated by instinctual pressure whose mental representation may take different forms. At the same time, psycho-analysts postulate fixation points to which the regressive movement retreats. These fixation points are the result of a failure in the developing capacity for object relationships in infancy and early childhood. According to these theories, when the schizophrenic patient confronts the clinician he does so equipped with a mental state nearer to that of the young infant than of the grown adult. The cognitive deficiencies and other symptoms that characterize the patient's mental state can thus be crudely equated with this infantile mental condition. It is not considered to be equivalent to or identical with a specific developmental phase but to contain within it important features which belong to the infantile period, as well as remnants of later and more advanced mental processes. A return to this primitive state (regression) enables the patient to avoid awareness of unwanted mental contents belonging to adult life.

The regression to an infantile phase of mental development implies that the mental processes employed to meet instinctual demands will then operate once more. This is a view taken by the followers of Melanie Klein. They see the phenomena of the schizophrenias as in part the outcome of a revival of mental mechanisms which have been relegated to a minor role in the mental economics of the healthy adult. The withdrawal, negativism, unresponsiveness, and inability to attend are regarded as the result of special forms of object relationship (transference psychosis) and not merely as the result of regression to an autoerotic, objectless phase, as the classical psycho-analytic theory would have it. According to these investigators (Rosenfeld; Bion) the above-mentioned phenomena represent the outcome of an attempt to banish the dread of a destructive hate originally directed against the mother's breast and body by means of mechanisms which ordinarily operate in infancy. The clinical manifestations result, first, from a projection of destructive phantasies into the clinician and, second, from splitting mechanisms whereby parts of the infantile ego that are contaminated by destructive phantasies are pushed into the object (the clinician). This is the mechanism conceptualized as projective identification. Processes of internalization (introjection) lead to the incorporation of the projected splits, thus leading to persecution from within. These defences (Rosenfeld, 1952) lead to the patient's negativism and to his tendency to confuse himself with others, to his dread of loss of identity, and to an inability to relate meaningfully to the environment.

Bion (1957) has elaborated this hypothesis further in an attempt to explain the cognitive disturbances prominent in the schizophrenias. He believes that a splitting of all those mental processes which will later constitute the ego organization – attending, thinking, perceiving, and remembering – takes place as a means of ridding awareness of both external and internal reality. This fragmentation results from the hatred of a reality which has proved so unsatisfying. The fragments are then expelled and projected into both animate and inanimate objects. The 'particles' may even engulf the objects, which then lead an independent existence. This process of projective identification leads to the patient experiencing his own cognitive functions as emanating from the environment.

In this approach (Bion, 1957), the fragmentation of cognition which obstructs effective communication with both self and the environment is conceived of as being the result of attempts to neutralize fear and hate of outer and inner worlds. In the clinical situation the infantile mechanisms of defence reassert themselves. Whatever verbal transactions may arise are fragmented and projected as a consequence of the destructive hatred along with the mechanisms of splitting and projective identification. In this way the affective accompaniments of an interpersonal relationship are avoided — expectations, demands, and fears of disappointment and loss are denied entry to consciousness. As Bion (1958) puts it, the schizophrenic patient substitutes primitive defences of the infantile period for the repression that would be employed by the healthy or psychoneurotic individual. The destructiveness also affects perceptual processes, leading to the interpenetration and equivalence of sensory modalities.

According to this theory, defects in the capacity for sustained attention result from the patient's unconscious unwillingness and inability to invest either the environment or the world of his thoughts with cathexis, for fear of affective and instinctual involvement. Hatred of objects and the defences against this make sustained attention impossible. A similar hypothesis is advanced by Searles (1959a), who does not adhere to the theoretical formulations regarding mental development proposed by Melanie Klein. He looks upon the dedifferentiation of cognition in the schizophrenias as a defence of a primitive kind. He believes, further, that the patient regards his cognition as something apart from himself belonging to the world of the persecutors.

These theories (Rosenfeld, 1952; Bion, 1957, 1958; Searles, 1961) are of great importance for psychotherapeutic work with schizophrenic patients because they give the therapist a means of understanding the psychotic behaviour and offer a mode of communicating which lays principal stress upon the fear and consequences of destructiveness which may arise in interpersonal relationships (see Chapter 10). Bion, Searles, and other authors give numerous examples of the manner in which cognitive functions alter in their expression parallel with changes in object relationships as evidenced within the patient-therapist situation. These relationships, as mentioned above, are always regarded by these authors as transferences, that is, as repetitions of real and phantasied experiences of infancy.

These hypotheses have been described in detail because they underline the fact that it is not enough merely to record the loss or the recovery of the capacity to attend and concentrate or to note the changes which may affect perceptual processes. These theories are important because they point to the possibility, often referred to by earlier writers (Bleuler; 1911; Sullivan, 1962), that these changes are secondary to interpersonal reactions. It would seem, therefore, that any serious study of cognitive function in the schizophrenias cannot be undertaken without special attention being given to the patient's past and current object relationships, especially to what transpires between the patient and the clinician. Psycho-analytic reports on the schizophrenias are well documented with illustrations of the parallel so often found between cognitive deterioration on the one hand and affective disturbance in the patient-physician relationship on the other hand (Freeman, 1962).

The theories which have been just described differ in many respects from the classical psycho-analytic view originally propounded by Freud (1911) and elaborated by others. In the former the schizophrenic phenomena are regarded as being the equivalent of a quasi-infantile form of object relationship and thus having a specific meaning in terms of phantasy content. The latter theory, however, does not acknowledge such specificity. According to this approach, the cognitive dysfunction is due to the ego regression, which leads among other consequences to the intrusion of the primary process. It is this form of mentation, with its condensations, displacements, and preference for concrete, pictorial representation, which leads to the disruption of conceptual thinking and of perceiving and to an inability to selectively attend. Though these phenomena can be related to anxiety and guilt arising out of inter-personal conflicts, they are not thought of as having specific phantasy content. They will increase or decrease in extent according to the pressure exerted by such anxiety. They are, in effect, the expression of a mode of mental functioning which ordinarily appears only in dreams or in humour. In spite of this serious difference with regard to the interpretation of the psychotic phenomena, there is general agreement among psycho-analysts that the clinical data are completely dependent upon the vicissitudes of object relationships and that changes in the former will always follow the fluctuations of the latter. From a psychotherapeutic standpoint, all psycho-analytic authors are agreed that fundamentally the symptomatology of the schizophrenic patient represents a means of avoiding anxiety and guilt.

DEFENSIVE PROCESSES IN PSYCHOSIS

A further aspect of ego function now requires to be examined in some detail because it plays an important part in the construction, manifestation, and content of certain psychotic symptoms. This is the defensive functioning of the ego (see Chapter 8). Ego defences must be categorized as follows — first, those which are characteristic of the adult ego and, second, those which operate during early phases of ego development. The latter can be said to belong to the pre-ego period, if such a state can be envisaged as existing. Ego functioning begins, as Hoffer (1954) has pointed out, from the earliest months of life, even though these processes are unstable and in no way integrated. With the origin of ego functions comes the simultaneous appearance of the counter-cathectic barriers, which progressively limit the drives and the mechanisms that govern their functioning (the primary process) and permit access to such consciousness as exists.

Rapaport (1953) has suggested that with the growth of the ego there is an accompanying development of a series of thresholds which impose limits upon the expression of the instinct drives, their mental representations, and the affects. He has proposed that there is within the ego a hierarchy of thresholds which permit a fine regulation of energy expenditure, in contrast with the 'all-or-nothing' reaction of the id cathexes. It is this delicate control that underlies the capacity for environmental adaptation and finds expression in the mental processes of conceptual thought, perceptual constancy, memory schemata, and control of motility. These thresholds are essentially counter-cathexes operating with neutralized energy. Defects in their function may be the cause of the characteristic form which schizophrenic symptoms assume.

During the early stages of mental development, which are characterized by a weak discriminatory capacity between the ego and objects, and prior to the appearance of the superego, the defence against the drives is motivated primarily by the pleasure-pain principle. Defence is essentially an economic question, being set in motion whenever there is an accumulation of drive energy. The absence of a clear differentiation between the ego, on the one hand, and the id, on the other, leads to a situation where mechanisms which belong to the system Unconscious can be used for defensive purposes as discharge of drive energy is the principal aim. Displacement of cathectic energy is utilized as a defence, as is the reversal of an instinctual aim. Activity is replaced by passivity. Closely associated with this mechanism is the trend whereby a drive is turned in on the self. The latter may be regarded as the forerunner of introjection.

Introjection and projection arise initially as a means of assimilating and structuring environmental stimuli but they soon come to assume a defensive function. Introjection is based upon reversal of aim but it embraces simultaneously the interaction of subject and object. Introjection has as its forerunner the condensation mechanism of the primary process and in early ego phases introjection is facilitated by this mechanism. Both introjection and projection can come into operation only whenever the ego boundary has achieved some small degree of stability. Mention must also be made of regression as a pre-ego defence. Drive energy is converted into imagery which may have a hallucinatory quality and thus find a mode of discharge. Denial is yet another mechanism which operates in infancy and which can be compared with the phenomena of negative hallucination and sensory inattention.

The establishment of ego and superego marks the appearance of new and important defences – particularly repression and identification. Objects are firmly established within the ego as a result of identification and do not only have an ephemeral passage, as occurs when the internalization results from introjections at earlier ego phases. With the appearance of the superego, the introjective mechanism can turn aggressive drive energy away from objects and into the superego, thus increasing the punitive aspects of the latter. Projection also assumes a different quantity with the final development of the ego – no doubt due to the firm boundary separating the ego from the world of objects. The clinical facts suggest that there is a psychotic projection (see Chapter 8, 'Defence') which is compounded with denial mechanisms. Reaction formation is yet another process that is dependent upon the functioning of a mature ego.

The examination of psychotic patients of all kinds reveals different defence mechanisms operating adequately or being defective in their function (see Chapter 8). A rough and approximate parallelism exists between the degree of ego and superego disintegration, on the one hand, and the kind of defensive processes which occur, on the other. Patients with well-organized paranoid delusions reveal a failure of repression in the region of the delusions – the content of which is denied and projected. This failure leads to such contents as incestuous phantasies, homosexual preoccupations, and pregenital tendencies of all kinds. In such cases the ego and superego otherwise seem to be intact – the cognitive functions are not contaminated by the primary process and there is evidence only of a selective failure of the countercathectic barriers. Depressive manifestations may appear in these well-organized cases of paranoid schizophrenia as a consequence of introjection of aggressive drives into the superego, concomitantly there may be self-reproach and suicidal attempts as a result of the introjection of the hated objects into the ego. Isolation may help to dissociate any thought or affect from the person of the physician if the patient is in psychotherapeutic treatment.

The situation is different in certain acute and chronic psychotic reactions. In these cases the ego and the superego appear to have suffered serious deterioration, and this is evidenced in the extensive cognitive (ego) deterioration and the loss of self-object discrimination. Violent eruptions of instinct drive indicate a failure of the counter-cathectic barriers. Repression is completely in abeyance, the patient expressing and acting upon what were previously repressed phantasies — sometimes they find representation in grandiose delusions. Reversal of aim — the substitution of passivity for activity — is often seen, as are denial and displacement (see Chapter 8). Other mechanisms, particularly introjection — which is frequently observed — do not seem to have a specific defensive function. The patient seems to assimilate the object without any special purpose or aim. There is often no sign whatever of projection, and certainly reaction formations are notable by their absence.

Just as the ego has antecedent stages of development, so has the superego. Freud (1923) laid down a general hypothesis regarding this development process. It follows the oedipus complex and consists of an internalization of the parental figures. It thus has its origins in the id, from which object cathexes sprang. During the first phases of development, the precursors of the superego consist of the introjected phantasy objects, which may be projected or re-introjected. The change of location is facilitated by the unstable nature of the ego boundary which makes inner/outer discrimination difficult. The introjected and projected objects are affectively coloured by the predominating instinctual demands. The superego may become the recipient of much of the narcissism that characterized the early ego. This aspect of the superego was formerly categorized under the concept of the ego ideal. The greater the narcissism arising out of narcissistic fixation, the more unrealistic and grandiose become the standards which the superego insists upon, thus leading to considerable ego-superego tension. Heightened narcissism may therefore find expression via the superego and not directly, as occurs in the sexual deviations. Consideration must be given to the possibility that this particular form of narcissism and the mode of its representation is to be distinguished from psychotic narcissism (Freeman, 1963, 1964).

AFFECT THEORY IN PSYCHOSIS

Some light may be thrown on the affective disturbance in schizophrenic states by reference to the affective reactions which occur in dreams. The affects in these two classes of phenomena are frequently characterized by being inappropriate or of low intensity. When affects occur in dreams, however, they give an indication of the trend of the latent dream thoughts. In this respect they are more reliable than the ideational material of the manifest content. As Freud says (1900), 'Analysis shows us, that the ideational material has undergone displacements and substitutions, whereas the affect remains unaltered'. In this regard, dreams show a most striking resemblance to schizophrenic states. In such patients anger or depression may seem to be completely out of keeping with the accompanying ideational content, but an examination of the total psychical situation will show that the affective reaction is appropriate. Anna Freud's (1936) remarks on the importance of affects in child analysis are particularly relevant for the study and treatment of schizophrenic patients whose capacity for intelligible verbal communication is impaired. As with children, excessive reliance on symbols— plentiful are they are — can be very misleading. The affects provide a more reliable index of the patient's mental state. This is essentially what Anna Freud (1936) says in the following quotation: 'It is therefore a fact of peculiar importance in child analysis, that, in observing the affective processes, we are largely independent of the child's voluntary co-operation and his truthfulness or untruthfulness in what he tells us. His affects betray themselves against his will.'

In his discussion of the cause of suppression of affect in dreams, Freud (1900), suggests the possibility that this phenomenon is due to a weakening of the processes underlying affects in much the same manner as motor impulses are inhibited during sleep. If this was true then ' . . . the affective impulses occurring during the course of the dream thoughts would from their very nature be weak impulses and consequently those which found their way into the dream would be no less weak' (Freud, 1900). This theory, Freud pointed out, would indicate that it was the state of sleep and not the dream-work which led to the suppression or weakening of affect. He rightly rejected this theory as far as dreams were concerned. It might, however, have relevance for schizophrenia if considered in conjunction with the withdrawal of cathexes from objects which occurs in these states.

Clinical observation, particularly during psychotherapy, leaves no doubt that the schizophrenic patient has a full range of affective re-actions at his disposal. Deviation from normality occurs in the control of the affects and their association with inappropriate behaviour and verbal communication. The understanding of the phenomenon of weakening of affects is complicated by the fact that there is an inade-quate distinction made between this phenomenon and withdrawal of interest (object cathexes) in the objects of the environment – the latter may easily be mistaken for the former. For example, a young woman of twenty-seven was admitted to hospital some three months after the birth of her second child. She was completely apathetic and with-drawn. She replied to all questions with the phrase 'I don't know'. She had no awareness of her name, her age, whether she was married or single, or where she lived. She met all inquiries with a blankness of expression or a look of bewilderment. She had so withdrawn her interest from the world that she was unresponsive to requests – to sit down, to recognize familiar objects, and so on. She would continue standing when offered a seat and she had to be spoon-fed. In spite of this pronounced and obvious withdrawal of cathexes from objects and from the ego functions, she was still capable of an affective response. On at least two occasions tears began to pour down her face accompan-ied by indisputable signs of despair – she said 'Oh God', but nothing further. Two days later she expressed her loss of contact with the world in this statement – 'No feeling, no head, no thoughts, no noth-ing.' Her emotional reaction consisted of an outburst of tears and the question, 'What is happening to me?' A few minutes later she said, 'Please I want to die.' In this case there was a withdrawal of cathexes from objects but the capacity for affective expression was retained. In many cases withdrawal of cathexes (interest in objects) is mistakenly identified with affective blunting.

Rapaport's (1953) comprehensive review and provisional statement of the psycho-analytical theory of affects underwrites this clinical distinction between withdrawal of cathexes and affect disturbance. He reminds his readers that in the first (cathartic) phase of psycho-analysis affect was equated with the quantity of psychic energy, which was later described as drive cathexis. He points out that even today there is a tendency among psycho-analysts to refer to affects as though they were identical in their nature with psychic energy. The fact is that, as early as 1900, Freud had thrown aside this theory and substituted the con-ception of affects as psychic formations distinguishable from drive cathexes. Affects, like ideas, are drive representations – safety valves which permit the release of accumulated drive cathexes which have been denied immediate discharge.

Rapaport suggests that, with the development of the ego, the affects partially abandon their safety-valve function and come to assume the role of signals. This 'taming' process (Rapaport, 1953) is achieved by the appearance of discharge thresholds which progressively inhibit the expression of affect. Such hypotheses provide an explanation for some of the affective disturbances in schizophrenic states. In those conditions the affects have lost their role as signals — the patient is unresponsive to dangers or to stimuli which would lead to grief or joy in the healthy individual. When they make their appearance they are characterized by an intensity and a transience which is more appropriate to the role of a safety valve indicating the presence of accumulated drive cathexes.

MELANCHOLIA AND MANIA

This account of the psycho-analytic theory of psychosis and the concepts which forms an integral part of it cannot be concluded without some comments on the illnesses variously described as melancholia, psychotic depression, or manic-depressive psychosis. Those patients who fall ill with this condition would appear to have developed, in the pre-psychotic period, a narcissistic disposition which influences them to make object choices of a narcissistic kind. In such instances the choice is made according to the standards set up by the superego (ego ideal). Disappointment in or loss of the object leads to a narcissistic regression.

Every case of depression does not regress to a psychotic narcissism as in the other functional psychoses. Not every patient reverts to an omnipotence of thinking or to the pathological egocentrism which is characteristic of other psychotic states. In all instances there is a withdrawal from objects and their representations, but this varies from one case to the next. It is most profound in those patients where the regression to a psychotic narcissism takes place. In those who regress to a non-psychotic narcissism, preoccupation with the self is uppermost, but the self is not the centre of all mental and environmental occurences. In psychotic depressions, the introjection into the ego of the lost or disappointing object and identification with it can be seen and may be regarded as a restitutional tendency. This introjection is not so obvious in those who are less severely disturbed. The inappropriate self-reproaches which occur in all true depressive states support this theory of introjection.

Withdrawal from objects, regression, and introjection leading to identification appear to be the main mechanisms in depressive reactions.

Freud regarded a large category of the functional psychoses, including the paranoid psychoses and melancholia, as narcissistic neuroses and compared them with the transference neuroses. Although the term 'neurosis' is confusing when applied to a psychotic reaction, the concept is an important one because it draws together many conditions that do not fit at all easily into the nosological concepts employed at the present time (see Chapter 8). Cases in point are those which show a mixture of paranoid and depressive manifestations — the so called schizo-affective states. At the same time, the narcissistic neuroses can be distinguished sharply by a number of criteria from the schizophrenic reactions. According to the classical theory, narcissistic neuroses are conditions in which the essential psychopathological process consists of a breakdown (regression) of the instinctual basis of object relations, which leads to a psychotic narcissism. In such cases the ego remains almost wholly intact. The sense of identity is retained, cognitive processes function at a good level, and hallucinatory phenomena do not appear. They are, however, characterized by delusional ideas and a pathological egocentrism which leads to a misinterpretation of perceptual experience (see Chapter 8).

It will not have escaped notice that no reference has been made to manic reactions and, indeed, little will be said about them. These cases which show extensive cognitive dysfunction along with over-activity and delusional ideation need not be manic reactions. Denial and repression of depressive affects would appear to be the main mechanisms at work in the uncomplicated manic state. Complex pathological theories which see the manic attack as representing the triumph over and killing of an internalized object may be merely exploiting thought contents which only some patients reveal. The content of what one patient reveals does not entitle the observer to generalize this into a hypothesis regarding the essential mechanism of the mental state. The presence of oral, anal, oedipal, or destructive phantasies does not differentiate one psychotic state from another, since these contents can be found in psychoses which are, on phenomenological grounds, entirely different in nature. They occur in organic psychoses (Gillespie, 1963). Classification of phenomena can be undertaken by reverting to the concepts that designate the mental processes envisaged as operating in the functional psychoses. Content must always remain secondary to this, even though this content may give a pointer to the specific endopsychic stresses that may have initiated the pathological processes.

CHAPTER 3

Psycho-analytic Technique as an Investigation Procedure

An essential component of research in the psychoses is the provision of a means of eliciting the patient's subjective experiences. This is a difficult task, because the patient does not consider himself ill or recognize the significances of his abnormal mental experiences. The patient will not purposively direct the psychiatrist's attention to his disturbed functioning, as will a patient who suffers from a physical ailment. A greater demand is therefore made upon the psychiatrist to find a method that will assist him in reaching the clinical phenomena. Though psycho-analysis is not the only psychological theory to offer a clinical technique that can be employed with psychotic patients, it has the advantage of emphasizing the pronounced resistances that characterize patients suffering from abnormal mental states. This warns an investigator that the patient will not easily unburden himself, even though he may be consciously willing to do so. Psycho-analysis also regards every aspect of a patient's behaviour as a potential communication. In this chapter the way in which psycho-analytic technique can be used as a means of investigating psychotic patients will be described. The problems that arise during such an undertaking will also be discussed.

It is impossible to overemphasize the need for detailed clinical description in research projects dealing with psychotic states. Eminent research workers have pointed out that many studies have turned out to be valueless because there was no clear indication of the patient's mental state at the time of the investigation or immediately prior to it. Winder (1961) and King & Rabin (1959) have stated that psychological investigations into psychotic states will never produce valid results until they are accompanied by a detailed statement of the patient's clinical status. Only such descriptions will permit the comparison of one study with another. Psychiatrists are well aware that the concept of schizophrenia or of manic-depressive psychosis does not have the same meaning for every clinician. It is not enough for those who study psychotic states to refer to their material mainly by diagnostic categories. It is essential for research workers to present details of the symptomatology and of cognitive dysfunctions which appear in the individual case. These data can be recorded in different ways. First, there is the time-honoured method of writing an account of the interview after it has been completed. Second, it is possible to use rating scales. In order to offset the vagueness engendered by the sole use of nosological concepts, it is preferable to describe the form of psychotic symptoms and behaviour and whatever fluctuations occur in their expression within the context of the patient-physician situation.

Since Jung (1907), Bleuler (1911), and Freud (1911) published their pioneering studies on the psychoses, psycho-analysis has been regarded as the theoretical model which best provides explanations for the clinical phenomena and a technique whereby these data may be elicited. Many authors – beginning with Schilder (1923) and Federn (1949) – have pointed out why the classical psycho-analytical method is inapplicable to cases of schizophrenia and have recommended various alterations in technique. In more recent times some psycho-analysts have even maintained that it is possible to apply the classical technique to patients suffering from schizophrenia.

The psycho-analyst who is engaged in the investigation or treatment of psychotic patients is primarily concerned with getting the patient to improve his capacity for communication and to widen and deepen the awareness of his psychological experiences. In this respect the psycho-analyst does not differ from the psychiatrist who bases his approach on the school of phenomenology. The psycho-analyst, like the phenomenologist, is continuously concerned with obtaining a complete description of the patient's subjective experiences. Only when this is obtained does the psycho-analyst attempt to relate these phenomena to the patient's life experiences, to his phantasy reactions, and to his responses to the physician. There is, in fact, no clash between the psycho-analytic approach and that of the clinical psychiatrist who sets out to discover as much as he can about the psychotic patient's experiences of his symptoms. It would seem that the psycho-analyst wants to go further than this and find a meaning for these mental experiences and, while doing so, to try to understand the way in which they have come about and why they have assumed their particular form.

The psycho-analyst, in common with the phenomenologist, recognizes the changing nature of psychotic symptomatology, but he is inclined to regard these changes as related to the patient's interpersonal reactions. Current interpersonal reactions are regarded by psycho-analysts as the stimuli which lead to alterations in symptoms and behaviour. In the special context of research, the question of therapy does not arise. The investigator is solely interested in finding out as much as he can about the patient's subjective experience. Psycho-analysis provides a technical framework whereby this may be achieved. Though this does not mean the employment of the psycho-analytic method as used in the treatment of the neuroses, it implies the utilization of such basic technical concepts as unconscious resistance and transference. The coming together of patient and physician implies the inevitable presence in some degree of processes conceptualized by these terms.

TECHNICAL AND THEORETICAL ASPECTS OF
PSYCHO-ANALYSIS

Too often what is unique to the psycho-analytic method is obscured by subsidiary considerations. The psycho-analytic method is characterized by a special concern for the details of the patient's behaviour in the clinical setting. The psycho-analyst is primarily interested in finding out the patient's preferred behavioural patterns as they are revealed in his utterances or in his actions. Only when they are identified is he in a position to search for the stimuli which possibly operate as activators of such patterns. The question of interpretation — what these behavioural manifestations mean and how they came to appear — has become a controversial issue both among psycho-analysts and among those who hold other views. It is the attention to detail that most characterizes the psycho-analytic method and in so doing offers the clinician a particularly good instrument for clinical investigation, despite the many difficulties and unknowns existing in this area. A brief glance at some fundamental psycho-analytic concepts is necessary in order to illustrate the manner in which the method may be helpful in studying the psychoses.

The psycho-analyst has a twofold aim when he initiates a psycho-analytical treatment in a case of neurosis. He hopes to understand the origin and mechanism of the illness and simultaneously to relieve the patient of his symptoms. Such a favourable outcome is to be expected in well-selected cases. Psycho-analysis combines therapeutic and scientific aims. Some years ago Rickman (1948) coined the aphorism 'no research without therapy, no therapy without research'. The formal requirements of the psycho-analytic method demonstrate the value which is laid upon the scientific aspects of the procedure. The expectant attitude of the psycho-analyst, the permissive atmosphere of the treatment situation, and the basic rule of free association allow him to observe, in the best possible circumstances, the form and content of the patient's utterances and behaviour.

The therapeutic orientation of the psycho-analytic method, however, interferes with its scientific aim. This is only one aspect of the matter; another is the appearance of unconscious resistance. Such resistance can block the emergence of clinical material. It is for this reason that the psycho-analyst must sometimes intervene. These interventions have a positive value, not least being the way in which links are forged between isolated and apparently disconnected ideational complexes. In this way the psycho-analyst helps the patient to adopt an inquiring attitude to his own mental contents. This is an essential prerequisite for a successful analytic undertaking, and its lack in psychotic states gives rise to extreme difficulty in communication.

A conflict between the need to cure and the need to understand is constantly in the psycho-analyst's mind. It is the latter need which helps him to withstand the temptation to exploit the magical (suggestive) elements which are intrinsic to every patient-therapist relationship. By resisting this temptation to omniscience and omnipotence, he is given the opportunity to examine and sometimes understand the nature and quality of the patient's interpersonal relationships.

The scientific approach demands that phenomena be observed in their natural setting. This is a counsel of perfection in the study of mental illness, since the psycho-analytic setting, in common with any other clinical situation, can be only partially observed and recorded. The psycho-analyst cannot, as in the case of a physical scientist, put down his material at will and take it up again at another time when he may be less fatigued, and thus more reliable in his recording capacity. At the beginning of the treatment the psychiatrist or psycho-analyst is without knowledge of the multiplicity of variables which activate the patient's responses. Initially he dare not emulate the detachment and objectivity of the biologist or physicist if he wishes to retain the object of his inquiries. He finds himself forced to participate, however minimally, in the relationship. His interventions which have a therapeutic aim (interpretations) may have adverse as well as beneficial effects. They may interfere with the order of the emerging phenomena and seriously influence the content of the patient's thinking. It is not uncommon for patients in a state of positive transference or in resistance to bring the kind of content which they think will please or annoy the psycho-analyst.

The psycho-analyst is in the difficult position of having to set up hypotheses that provide an explanation of the patient's behaviour. Many of these hypotheses have to be discarded as valueless. He recognizes that at best what he will present to the patient is not an exact reproduction of the latter's conflict but only an approximation to it. In optimal circumstances the psycho-analyst will refrain from proposing explanations which are not easily extracted from the observable phenomena. It is always necessary to bear in mind that the presentation of interpretations is a vital part of the analyst's therapeutic task and is often necessary to keep the patient in the analytic situation.

An interpretation is a specific form of communication whose aim is either to present information to the patient of which has he been previously unaware or to join together isolated ideational contents. Interpretations can be broadly divided into two classes. First, there are those which are directed to unconscious contents and, second, there are those which are directed at the analysis of resistances. In a sense this division is an artificial one, because the analysis of resistances leads to the exposure of specific unconscious contents.

The interpretations most likely to interfere with the scientific aim of the psycho-analysis, i.e. the understanding of the patient's illness, are those which are concerned with unconscious content. Castration wishes, oedipal rivalry, and anal-sadistic phantasies are good examples of this. However, it is easy to exaggerate this difficulty if psychoanalytical interpretation is regarded as a form of indoctrination whereby the patient is presented with concrete statements regarding his wish to destroy or fear of destroying the transference object, his fear of castration, and so on. In psycho-analytic therapy these phantasies are interpreted initially in their derivative forms, which are far distant from their infantile, bodily origins. Later, the patient may be able to discern their basic nature himself.

When a patient is confronted with interpretations he may, depending upon his personality, find himself no longer presenting his own ideas but rather employing the language of the analyst. Such behaviour must be regarded as a legitimate phenomenon arising out of the inter-action between patient and analyst and requiring examination as would any other form of resistance. This material must be scrutinized to see what purpose it serves. That is what happens in the psycho-analytical therapy of the neuroses. Unfortunately, the effect of inter-pretation on the psychotic patient is much more difficult to assess, and on this ground alone there seems a case to limit such communications to a minimum if understanding of the patient's problem is regarded as the primary aim.

In certain phases of psycho-analytic treatment interpretation of repressed content is an important and essential step. However, it is just this kind of interpretation which has led to so much disagreement among psycho-analysts and non-analysts. Among the former, there are many who believe that certain contents (oral-sadistic phantasies, persecutory fears) must be given priority in interpretation. The latter, on the other hand, equally express scepticism regarding the validity of these contents and look upon the effect of the interpretations as com-pletely non-specific and not related to their content. However, these controversies are not immediately relevant in the present context.

Much of the disagreement centring upon interpretation of uncon-scious contents does not apply so forcibly to interpretation of resistances. The latter interpretations are solely concerned with the dissipation of unconscious tendencies which may disrupt the treatment relationship. They are less inferential and more phenomenologically based than interpretations of unconscious content. If the patient is allowed to express himself freely, patterns of reactions emerge which are in-appropriate to the analytic situation. Freud suggested that these re-actions are displaced from current or past situations into the treatment room and onto the person of the psycho-analyst.

Interpretations of transference resistance which are based upon 'here-and-now' phenomena are of the greatest importance in main-taining the viability of a psycho-analytic treatment and enabling the patient to bring new material. Much of the psycho-analytic process consists of transference interpretations. These interpretations are based upon careful observation of the patient's utterances and behaviour in the treatment room. With a psycho-neurotic patient, interpretation of resistances will often lead to new material which helps further understanding. There is no guarantee of this with the psychotic patient, whose response may be quite incomprehensible even when the interpretation or reconstruction may have been approximately correct. It is necessary, therefore, in dealing with psychotic patients, to concentrate upon their behaviour and utterances in the clinical setting in the hope that this will eventually reveal some form of organization. In certain psychotic states interpretation is much more likely to obscure than clarify the processes going on in the patient's mind. The only exceptions to this general rule are those occasions where the patient becomes caught up by a fear of the analyst and threatens to break off the contact.

When approaching a psychotic patient, the psycho-analyst is faced with a number of problems which preclude a complete application of the psycho-analytical method. This has had the result of causing many psycho-analysts to doubt whether there is such a thing as the psychoanalytic therapy of the psychoses. They point out that the illness interferes with the patient's judgement, with the consequence that he does not regard himself as ill. Hence his capacity for co-operative work is limited. Frequently the patient is unable or unwilling to abide by the rule of free association. He sees no reason why he should attend daily or lie on a counch. This is true of the majority of patients who require hospitalization.

In view of these considerations, it is possibly more suitable to refer to the psycho-analytic approach to the psychoses as a form of psychoanalytical psychotherapy – that is, a psychotherapy which employs and adapts the principles of psycho-analytical treatment as used in the neuroses. The problems which the psycho-analyst faces with the psychotic patient are no less when the aim is one of data collection.

In the psycho-analytic treatment of the neuroses the psycho-analyst hopes to create those conditions which will promote the development of a transference neurosis and not simply the transference of current attitudes, expectations, and affects. The distinction between transference and transference neurosis is not an academic one. Every individual unconsciously displaces reactions from one person to another during his daily life. In psycho-analysis or analytic psychotherapy these displacements – 'floating' transferences to use Glover's (1955) expression – can be clearly observed. Transference is non-specific because it does not demonstrate a point-for-point correspondence between the original (infantile) object and the transference object. It can almost be regarded as a diffuse reaction response to the person of the physician.

At the beginning of the treatment much of the patient's reaction to the psycho-analyst is based on the reality aspects of the patient-doctor relationship. The transference neurosis gradually develops and its manifestations are specific for the individual when they appear within the psycho-analytical situation. It is a reaction which contains little of the real situation and is the result of the repetition of the content of childhood relationships. The patient repeats the various responses which he had to the objects of his childhood, only now directed to the person of the analyst.

The patient becomes extremely sensitive to the smallest and least perceptible aspect of the analyst's behaviour. While non-specific transference reactions which appear at the outset of therapy have infantile roots, they cannot be recognized nor do they have significance for the patient until the psycho-analyst becomes important in the patient's emotional life. The psycho-analyst always hopes that during the treatment of a neurosis non-specific transferences will gradually be replaced by a transference neurosis.

The recumbent position, the psycho-analyst out of sight, and free association lead in favourable instances to a regression of the temporal variety described by Freud (1955). Psychical reality is enhanced at the expense of current reality. Thinking becomes permeated by affective attitudes appropriate to childhood and thus the repetition of childhood object relationships is facilitated (the transference neurosis). Only a part of the patient's ego is affected by this regression. He is always able to reflect upon what he is experiencing and can make some form of rational criticism. In this way he can accept or reject interpretations which are directed towards the analysis of the transference neurosis. When the patient leaves the analytic couch there is a tendency for the regression to disappear. This will not happen in patients who suffer from severe neuroses, from addictions, and from borderline states. Such patients may regress too far in the treatment situation and often they cannot control the effects of this process. They often present very difficult problems of management both within and outside the analytic hour. Interpretation does not always have a reassuring effect nor does it lead to therapeutic improvement.

PROBLEMS ENCOUNTERED IN PSYCHOSIS

In the psychoses the situation is much more complicated because the clinician is dealing with a patient whose personality structure is severely damaged. How does this damage affect technique in general and specifically how does it affect the development of the transference neurosis? This is indeed the crucial question, because a patient's capacity to participate and his amenability to therapeutic influence are entirely dependent upon the availability of 'genuine' transferences whose origin is in the childhood period. All psycho-analysts agree that schizophrenic patients are capable of some kind of object relationship. Reference was made in Chapter 2 to the concept of transference psychosis, which is employed by some psycho-analysts to describe the psychotic patient's relationship to the psycho-analyst whatever form it may assume. This concept — transference psychosis — is useful in a practical sense because it describes constellations of clinical phenomena, but it should be distinguished sharply from the genuine transferences which are essential for therapeutic influence. Transference psychotic phenomena are not 'genuine' transferences but are analogous to the 'floating' or spontaneous transferences referred to earlier.

It is often difficult to identify with confidence psychotic phenomena as aspects of a transference neurosis — that is, as repetitions of childhood object relationships. All that can be said is that the patient reacts to the analytic situation, but the nature of the reaction is complex, made up of many unknown factors springing from the current situation, the symptomatology, the clinical situation, and the past — this always including the contribution of unconscious phantasies.

(a) Disturbances of Identity and Sense of Self

There are many patients who demonstrate a defect in the integrity of the sense of identity. The true identity is often denied and replaced by another identity. In some cases the new identity remains constant over many years. This identity is sometimes valued by the patient and at other times resented because of the belief that it has been imposed upon him. In these cases the patient is constantly in a state of confusion because he cannot discriminate between his old identity and the new one. There are patients in whom the sense of identity alters in accordance with whomever they may be in contact with. The patient will assume the name and occupation of the person. If the patient is in contact with a doctor he is that doctor, if an attendant then he is that attendant, and so on. This tendency is often accompanied by a tendency to assimilate environmental stimuli, and it is this assimilation which determines the content of speech.

The extent of this assimilatory process varies between patients.

CASE 1. In the following verbatim statement obtained from a patient suffering from hebephrenic schizophrenia, this trend was easily seen. 'What are you thinking about?' *Patient:* 'We have to wash and dry the dishes after breakfast . . .' Silence . . . 'Why are you silent?' *Patient:* 'I just sat down when you told me. By rights I should be going home. There is nothing wrong with me. I was only here to see someone else. They gave me a job. There was some suggestion it was a hospital. I was living at home. But my father is dead now . . . that's why you can say he's probably decided to smoke a pipe (the interviewer was smoking a pipe). They put the family in hospital . . .' He was reminded that he had said that his father was dead and he replied, 'He died out in Australia . . .' He was asked how his father could smoke a pipe if he was dead. *Patient:* 'He cannot do it now, he threatened to go into hospital . . . you get the answer after smoking a pipe . . . my father's smoking a pipe . . . he couldn't be bothered with you in the house but he is dead now . . .' 'He's a Freemason (similarity to the interviewer's name) . . . I heard of a case before of a man who couldn't smoke with his family in the house because someone barred against it. He put them out you see . . . he could stay a Freemason during his lifetime but he couldn't be buried as one . . . this man that is smoking his pipe — your brother could start doing the same thing . . . the man who put his family out wasn't living as a Freemason . . . he lived as a Freemason but he wasn't buried as a Freemason.'

This process of assimilation is probably due to faulty ego-boundary functioning, but in many cases, such as that quoted above, the patient did not fail to discriminate between himself and others. The capacity to discriminate between subject and object can be retained even though the identity aspects of the self-representation are unstable. On the other hand, identity problems and a defect in self-object discrimination can be found in the same patient. Here the patient attributes thoughts, sensations, and attitudes of his own to the physician and vice versa. Sometimes the discriminatory failure is best seen in the patient's behaviour and at other times in the patient's utterances, as in the following example.

CASE 2. In this case, a psychotic patient, there was a combination of penetration of the self into objects and objects into the self. Ideas were concretized and regarded as things by the patient. The assimilatory tendency was also present. The interviewer was wiping his glasses, having just asked the patient if she could tell him about her feelings. She replied, 'Yes I have, do you mean the feelings of cleaning your glasses so that you can see through them . . . that kind of feeling do you mean? Cleaning glasses so that you can see clear. I don't wear glasses but I could do with some. I've got too much sight, you may not have enough sight, I've got too much.' When asked to clarify this statement, she said, 'I've got the sight which can see the whole television at once, I feel as if I've got the whole light instead of a little light, just like looking through the window, just now you can see the whole building at once, I'm talking about sight for reading, you can see the whole page of the book, but I can't keep my mind to myself, they listen to everything I read.'

She continued: 'That means I can go right through you like that, that means I can look at you and go right through your brain and come back out again and you wouldn't know I was in there.' When asked how she could do that she said, 'I can, I'm a brain specialist just like the thin air, just like the light next door (referring to a test which she had just completed). I wish I was there and could show you what I mean — you've got a man's voice telling you about evil and things — is it a test to see if you are religious or something . . . ?' She was reminded that she had said that the light had gone into her head and come out again. She replied, 'That's true, yes, that's what he keeps doing to me, he goes right through me or thinks he's there, whatever he's supposed to be doing, a part of him is there, feelings of his own, he ought to keep them.' Did she mean that the psychologist's feelings were going into her today? 'Yes of course I do, you've got to shove them out.' When asked what the feelings were she said, 'Love, you can't say love feelings, you can't have love feelings, you could have kind feelings.' 'What is the red light you see when you keep switching on and off? What is the red light? Is it a torch bulb? I can do the same, I could push something in that you wouldn't know was there such as kindness for instance, speech, you have got kindnesss and you haven't much speech, you could call me a dumb blond if I didn't speak, no you haven't got very much speech you are a fairly quiet person and I am a quiet person if either of us didn't speak we're in between.'

She was asked what feelings had been pushed into her and she said, 'Just his own feelings, love feelings, love feelings which he has got and which he thinks I've got, yet he can do that, I can do that, but I've got to keep it for myself and smoke cigarettes, I like to have feelings of my own, some people wish they were me, every pain you can think of and everyone around about wanted to be like me because they thought I could sing and dance, speak, be a doctor, a nurse or a nun or anything I wish because I know how, I know how to be all these things, I know how to be you sitting there because I am you just now, I could be you just now because you are recording my voice and you will only get two words that is anything good if you are testing people's feelings and you push your feelings into me, it isn't me you're diagnosing it is yourself, it is himself not me, I am diagnosing you with that cigarette smoking, if you left it alone you could speak, you are too comfortable.' In this illustration the patient had lost the capacity to discriminate herself clearly from the person of the physician and this led to much confusion on the patient's part. It is a condition quite different from anything encountered during the psycho-analysis of a neurotic patient.

Psycho-analysis and analytical psychotherapy are essentially concerned with helping patients to re-experience the object relationship conflicts of the past and thus lead to a resolution of symptoms. In the neuroses, interpretation is the principal method used by the psychoanalyst to give the patient knowledge about the unconscious conflicts which lie at the root of his symptoms. The efficacy of interpretation is always dependent upon a transference which, in psycho-analytic terminology, is object-libidinal in nature. The patient is thus willing to consider the interpretation out of regard for the analyst – this prevents an immediate rejection of the latter's communication. The initial reception of an interpretation is therefore dependent upon a positive relationship between patient and analyst. In many patients suffering from psychoses self-preoccupation limits any true relationship with the analyst or psychotherapist. There is in fact no real relationship – no real wish to please the psychotherapist and thus give attention and interest to what is said. Interpretations can become effective only when the capacity for object relationships is at least partially present.

A somewhat similar state of affairs is to be encountered in the psycho-analytic therapy of patients with character abnormalities and sexual deviations. In these cases a narcissistic transference makes its appearance in which the analyst becomes endowed with the patient's narcissism. This narcissistic transference operates as a resistance against the appearance of the real transference (the transference neurosis) which can be employed for therapeutic ends. The patient protects himself against the recognition of his relationship conflicts through idealization and identification with the analyst. It is only after the resolution of this narcissistic transference that conflicts appear within the patient-physician situation and become subject to analysis (Freeman, 1964).

(b) *Effectiveness of Interpretations*

Although the reactions to interpretation of psychotic and sexually deviant patients are often similar, it would be erroneous to equate the narcissistic organizations which underlie the clinical phenomena. In character abnormalities and sexual deviations, the narcissism is akin to the secondary narcissism associated with a level of mental development in which self-object discrimination is present and the ego (the secondary process), has reached its mature function. The narcissism of a large category of psychotic patients is a pathological variant of primary narcissism (Freeman, 1963) where mental activity is governed by the primary process. Later (see Chapter 5) examples will be given of patients whose delusional content demonstrates not only a narcissistic choice of delusional object but also the operation of the mechanisms of the primary process – condensation and displacement.

Where there are disturbances in the sense of identity and loss of self-object discrimination, the patient cannot clearly distinguish himself from the person of the physician, and this leads to much confusion on the patient's part. Therapeutic influence is possible in cases of neuroses only by virtue of the separate existence of the psycho-analyst in the patient's mind and the latter's (patient's) ability to distinguish the former (analyst) from the objects of the past which he may have transferred onto him. This is the case even with the narcissistic transferences of the character defect and the sexually deviant. The seriously disturbed psychotic patient has lost the capacity to make this discrimination, not only because of the confusion brought about by the merging process (condensation) but also on account of the lack of reflective awareness of the self. The psychotic patient cannot discriminate the clinician from himself nor the objects of the past from his own image or that of the clinician. It is likely that Freud was referring to this kind of data when he said that schizophrenic patients were not amenable to psycho-analytic therapy and that they did not develop 'working' transferences.

The impact and efficacy of interpretation will depend upon a patient's potential for transference based upon object-libidinal cathexes. This capacity cannot be gauged by the reactions (misidentifications; negativism; self-object discriminatory failure; persecutory ideas) which are described by the concept of 'transference psychosis'. In Chapter 10 Cameron distinguishes between negativism and 'genuine negative transference'. The greater the capacity for relationships characterized by interest and affectivity, the better may be the transference potential (Glover, 1954). A further obstacle to the effective employment of interpretations in cases of psychosis results from the cognitive disorganization so frequently encountered in these conditions. It is doubtful whether the patient's attentive capacity and his ability to comprehend verbal symbols are sufficiently intact for him to understand the content of interpretations.

(c) Transference Potential

Eliciting a psychotic patient's subjective experiences depends upon two factors which are basically related to one another. From a descriptive or phenomenological standpoint they can be identified, first, as the extent of the patient's accessibility (object relations potential) and, second, how far the mental processes necessary for verbal communication remain unimpaired by the disease. The psycho-analyst will describe the first factor as the patient's transference potential and the second as the extent of the non-psychotic residues or non-psychotic layer (Katan, 1954). He may even think that a better understanding is to be obtained by relating the patient's capacity to describe his experiences to the depth of the regression in the spheres of the ego organization, on the one hand, and the instinctual base of object relations, on the other hand.

All psychotic patients do not necessarily show a regression in both areas. In one case the ego organization may be affected, thus leading to a failure to create and utilize the means of verbal communication. In such a patient the regression may not have severely affected the object relationship capacity, thus enabling the patient to enter into a clinical relationship even although handicapped by difficulties in verbal expression. On the other hand, when the regression affects the object relationship capacity the patient may be utterly inaccessible, even though his ego organization – his cognitive capacity – is virtually intact. Many psychotic patients with persecutory delusions fall into the latter category.

The transference potential of a psychotic patient will be dependent upon the extent of the regression affecting the instinctual base of object relations. The greater the psychotic narcissism, the less the capacity for transference. No one can know at the outset what form the psychotic patient's transference will take – assuming that the patient shows some kind of reaction to the clinician. Often it is impossible to obtain any data which might throw light on this because the patient appears indifferent and withdrawn. Even in such cases, however, there is a potential for response, but this responsiveness is dependent upon the presentation of a stimulus specific for the patient.

In clinical encounters whose main object is the obtaining of information, the investigator can only hope that the patient will at least be prepared to enter into some kind of relationship, however superficial. The former can have no knowledge at the outset of how the latter will react even when he has consented to attend for interview. Psychoanalytic theory provides the observer with a series of hypotheses which can be employed in the clinical setting. He must appeal to that part of the patient's mind which is not involved by the illness. Interestingly enough, many patients are quite happy to have daily interviews even though they may insist there is nothing wrong with them. In such instances it is almost as if the patient recognizes that he is in fact mentally ill and in need of help.

Although the psycho-analytically trained observer will initially refrain from unnecessary comment, he must nevertheless go forward to meet the psychotic patient and encourage him to express himself as freely as possible. When this is successful it leads to the patient's giving detailed accounts of the delusional or hallucinatory experiences.

(d) Cognitive Disorganization

When a patient's communications are studied over a period of a few days it becomes apparent that the cognitive disorganization need not remain constant either during the one interview or from one interview to the next. Alterations may occur between disorganized thinking and perceiving, on the one hand, and normal cognition, on the other. It is not easy to identify the cause for such changes and it is very attractive to turn to the theory which sees the patient's anxiety as leading to this primitivization (regression) and disorganization of cognition. It is conceivable that the observer is confronted with a process which, though wakened by interpersonal contact, has no specific aim as has a psychoneurotic symptom, which is concerned with keeping special mental contents from consciousness.

A number of psycho-analytic observers have commented on the fact that the disorganization of thinking and verbal communication is often reversed with the appearance of anger. Why do patients become coherent and logical with the appearance of a strong affect? Is it because they become less afraid or is it because the apathy and indifference which dominate their mental activity are dissipated and they operate adequately once again? This would fit in with Schilder's concept of psychic drive (1928a) — that psychotic patients often lack the drive necessary to energize the cognitive functions.

The clinical data do not give unqualified support to the theory that the regression and disorganization can always be reversed when the patient is aroused emotionally or is preoccupied with a need which he must communicate. There are chronic schizophrenic patients who show that even when they are able to express themselves verbally the form and content of speech are far removed from those of normal people. It would seem that there are varying levels to which the ego regresses and different forms of disorganization. The extent to which the regression may be reversed depends not only upon the depth of the regression but also upon other factors affecting the ego function which are thus far unknown. It may be these latter factors which prevent the return of normal cognition. Can schizophrenic patients be classified in terms of how far the regression extends and whether or not the deteriorated cognition shows a trend towards the return of normal functioning? Such a consideration is independent of theories which try to explain the reasons for this fluctuation, although any explanation must depend upon a genetic or developmental conception of mental functioning.

Schilder's (1928a) concept of brain apparatus which governs specific functions can be of value here. According to this formulation (implied in the view presented above), mechanisms which compose the apparatus can be impaired in their function by psychological influences. When these influences cease the apparatus regains its normal activity. Organic alteration of the apparatus leads to a permanent loss of function.

The fact that patients whose speech is deteriorated can communicate normally when in the grip of strong emotions can find another interpretation. In Schilder's view (1928) psychological forces can also act upon an apparatus organically affected in such a way as to oppose the effects of the disease. Here the organic defect is opposed by the psychological factor. He points out that this is to be seen in cases of postencephalitis who lose their organic symptoms under the influence of emotion. When the emotion disappears the symptoms return. It is as if the psychological forces are not strong enough to counteract the organic change in the apparatus brought about by the disease. It would appear, therefore, that a return of normal speech function does not necessarily indicate the presence of intact verbal capacity inhibited in expression by psychological factors.

How much significance is to be given, then, to the deterioration in the capacity for verbal communication? It is only through speech that one can detect abnormalities of the thought processes. How far can these defects be taken as indices of cognitive deterioration? These disturbances of speech and thinking are sometimes rectified permanently or only for short periods. All psychiatrists who have worked for any time in a mental hospital know that there are patients whose utterances are incoherent and chaotic and who are yet capable of carrying out useful tasks in hospitals and looking after themselves (see Chapter 5). It is observations of this type that suggest that the disorder of speech and thinking should not be taken as an overall measure of cognitive dysfunction. It is also such phenomena that give backing to the theory that the disorganization of thinking is a defensive manoeuvre on the part of the patient to escape from the conflicts and dangers inherent in interpersonal relations. This is the view of those who follow Sullivan and Melanie Klein.

Hebephrenic patients present special difficulties because of the ease with which cognition deteriorates, and it is the investigator's task to follow the patient's mental processes as best he can, recognizing that anxiety may be a cause of the dysfunction. Some believe that interpretation of the anxiety stimulus may lead to improved cognitive activity – particularly in the sphere of attention and verbal communication. The following clinical excerpt illustrates the difficulty which cognitively disorganized patients present.

CASE 3. The patient was a young woman aged twenty years who was hospitalized on account of confusion of mind, pronounced withdrawal, delusional ideation, and cognitive dysfunction. The interview to be described was one of a series of daily interviews. The session occurred about two weeks after admission and was recorded on tape. When she sat down she looked at a tape-machine which was in the room but made no comment. After some minutes she was asked what she was thinking about. She said in a low voice, 'I am the empress of the world' – this was repeated three times. 'I was canonized as Saint Anne ... I like this place.' She became silent and when asked to speak said,

'I'm hungry — I can't eat.' She continued to cast glances at the tape-recorder but remained silent for some minutes. Eventually she said, 'I like the world — I like the world . . .' A minute or two later she continued, 'People are nice and that . . . kings and queens are wonderful . . . each hundred years it gets better.'

She was asked why she kept looking at the tape-recorder. She said, 'I am looking at the white . . .' She meant she was looking at the blotting-pad on the desk. She followed this incomplete phrase by, ' . . . a Scottish accent.' She was asked what she meant by this and she replied, 'I believe I have a Scottish accent and sometimes I have an English accent and sometimes an American and when I was listening to the television in Italy or in France I could read their lips.'

This material was of interest because the day before she had told the interviewer that he had an American accent. The reference to accents could also have referred to a thought about what her own voice sounded like on the recording-machine. As she fell silent she was asked what she was thinking about. 'At the brown table — it is quite big . . . it is very nice in a way and it is strong.' This was a further reference to the interviewer because on the day before she had said that one of his arms looked strong.

She was asked again what she was thinking about. Eventually she said, 'Well I like . . .' She repeated this and was silent for a while until she said, 'My face is rather odd at times.' It seemed to the interviewer as if she was taken up with thoughts of their (patient and the doctor) physiques which she had been referring to on the previous day. Eventually she continued, 'My face is rather odd at times.' As she did not continue with this she was asked in what way was it odd. This question was met with silence, but then she said, 'Well, I have a broad face.'

Interviewer: 'You find it difficult talking to me.' *Patient:* 'Yes, to a man.' When asked why, she replied, 'Well I always get worried about it . . .' After a pause she continued, 'I am thinking of Paisley. It is a nice town, it is quite warm. There are houses being built. They pull down houses there, and are building fifteen- and twenty-storey flats. I think in Scotland and Glasgow there are twenty-storey flats because people are so crowded in houses and they can't breathe . . . and . . . in Paisley during the winter-time in the flats, the heating, something went wrong . . . and the people didn't like it during the winter because Scotland is very crowded . . .'

The material quoted shows that the patient could not continue with a theme to its conclusion. She evaded questions concerning the recorder or the interviewer and substituted apparently irrelevant data. What was the cause of this? Was it merely indifference or did it have an unconscious motivation? Her subsequent utterances revealed an anxiety (? libidinal) about the interview and the recording. 'Queen Elizabeth II is depressed because . . . in Scotland, the Presbyterians, the non-Catholics, are trying to agree with Pope John because of mixed marriages. There is a lot of mixed marriages in Great Britain . . . the children can get on very well but some way they get out of it . . . of course a lot of them get out of it because there are many . . . mixed marriages . . . when the child is born some people say they are quite clever but many . . . five years old . . . in Britain they have from five year old to they are fifteen . . . fifteen. . . . You know children from five to fifteen there is a lot of them have to pass their test when they are eleven years old.' *Interviewer:* 'You think of this interview as a test.' 'Yes, a test of faith and loyalty and understanding. I see the recorder.'

When asked what she thought about the recorder she replied, 'To see if I'm insane.' *Interviewer:* 'Are you insane?' 'No I don't think so . . . I am intelligent. Yes . . . but . . . in Scotland and England they have a jury of twelve people. Maybe in England they have more. I don't know whether I have done the wrong thing or not. I think I'm quite good. I am having a test to see if . . . insanity someone who is not really right but when you are judged by a jury in Scotland or England you could be hanged. But now of course it is much more modern — you go to jail or to see a psychiatrist.' *Interviewer:* 'Are you not a little afraid?' *Patient:* 'Well, they always say that the world is either square or round or oval-shaped . . . In America they have spacemen. They don't call them spacemen. They are in orbit up in the sky.' She continued, 'I'm not frightened because I am happy here. I believe I'm Saint Anne . . . I am a saint because I am here to save the world from corruption.'

It was as if the patient was able for a moment or two to acknowledge fear and guilt. However this was quickly covered over by the reappearance of delusion of grandeur and the denial of anxiety with an upsurge once again of a defect in the capacity to communicate verbally. Although from a therapeutic standpoint little had been achieved, the interventions enabled the investigator to find out something about the patient's subjective experiences.

This patient demonstrated a difficulty which is often present during continuous clinical contact with hebephrenic individuals — namely that it is often impossible to say whether transferences are present or not. Withdrawal, misidentifications, the fragmentation of verbal expression, and the psychic inertia render the recognition or identification of transference patterns extremely difficult. Searles (1963a) has also commented on the difficulty of elucidating transference manifestation in patients of this type.

The unbiased clinician must often feel that if he were to make a transference interpretation it would be more in the nature of his own invention than an actual description of what is taking place in the patient's mind. Hebephrenic patients react in a general way to the clinician, but the diffuse nature of this reaction suggests that it is better to confine interpretations to general comments regarding the former's attitude to confiding in another person and to his anxieties about this. This approach is especially important if the clinician's main objective is to gather information rather than to be primarily therapeutic.

Many cognitively deteriorated patients will continue their clinical contact over a long period of time and this alone suggests that they have made some kind of attachment to the person of the clinician. It is nevertheless true that their participation is often passive rather than active because they will forget interviews or come at the wrong time, and, when they do arrive, they have to be constantly stimulated to communicate, a feature that was particularly pronounced in the patient described above.

In this respect the hebephrenic patient may be contrasted with those psychotic patients whose illness is characterized by persecutory delusions. The evasive activity suspected in the hebephrenic, which, it is suggested, manifests itself in verbal incapacity, is replaced in these patients either by an intense suspiciousness or by a frank dislike of any close personal contact. It is often difficult to define a transference pattern as one would do in a psychoneurotic patient. These patients may be willing to attend for regular interviews, but frequently the material is characterized by a repetition of delusional ideas and hallucinatory experiences. The patient remains quite apart from the clinician.

Psycho-analytic theory is useful again because it points out that the contents of the delusions are in a sense partly true and contain within them important phantasies and conflicts that the patient has experienced at some time in his life. Enabling the patient to express these irrational

E

ideas provides the investigator with important data. Sometimes the content of hallucinations and delusions which appear during the course of interviews may indicate something of what the patient thinks about the clinician and the meetings. In this way the patient can disown all responsibility for his thoughts. These phenomena support the idea that the patient fears the consequences of interpersonal relationships as he envisages them.

Here again the problem of interpretation is difficult, but for different reasons. In paranoid psychoses the patient is not hampered by inadequate verbal capacity. When he talks he does so appropriately and he can easily be followed. In some paranoid cases certain patterns in the patient's object relationships can be discerned which may have arisen in the present or from the past and could be considered as potential transferences. The problem with respect to the significance of these patterns is that the patient makes it painfully clear that he is quite indifferent to the clinician. It may be, as Searles (1963a) and Cameron (see Chapter 10) report, that after long periods of contact identifiable transferences from the childhood period do occur. There is, however, no evidence at the present time that psychotic phenomena which are displaced into the treatment relationship can always be dispersed through interpretation and replaced with ideation and affects that are appropriate to an interpersonal situation. From an information-gathering standpoint paranoid psychoses are sometimes the least accessible.

TRANSFERENCE IN PSYCHOSIS

The types of patient described so far are those in which the illness can only be described as severe and the prognosis poor. Perhaps they fall into the category conceptualized as nuclear schizophrenia or dementia praecox in the older terminology. There is a whole category of patients who show many of the signs of either a schizophrenic illness or a paranoid reaction, but who are nevertheless able to develop an affective relationship with the clinician from almost the beginning of the clinical contact. In many ways they show similarities to the psycho-neurotic patient, particularly because they are never indifferent to the person of the clinician. In these cases it seems correct to say that genuine, employable transferences come into being – transferences similar to the transference neurosis of the neurotic reaction. A case of this kind has been described by Davie (1963). In this instance the patient's mental state alternated between a predominantly neurotic condition and serious psychotic disorganization.

The rapidity with which the clinician will find his way into the patient's mental life will depend upon the capacity for transference as understood in the treatment of the neuroses. So called 'psychotic transferences' do not make for this development. They result from an attachment of the predominant delusional complexes to the clinician or consist of misidentifications, faulty discriminations, and negativistic behaviour (see Chapter 10).

The success of the investigational procedure depends as much on the patient as on the skill and experience of the clinician. The physician cannot evoke transferences if the patient has no capacity for such developments. The physician's technique must be directed towards providing the setting in which transferences and other material may arise. In this undertaking extensive interpretation is unnecessary beyond those interventions which let the patient know that the clinician is aware of the patient's anxieties about the interview situation. In spite of much theorizing over the past ten to fifteen years about the technique necessary for approaching the psychotic patient, everyone who works with these patients tries to contact the non-psychotic processes which remain active within them. This is similar to Federn's (1948) approach in which primary emphasis was put upon the cultivation of a positive relationship with the patient. Federn knew that once persecutory ideas or a massive withdrawal characterized the interview situation little could be done to influence the patient. His observations are no less true today.

It is necessary to examine in greater detail the reaction of psychotic patients to the offer of an interpersonal contact. The patient's response throws some light upon the extent and availability of his object cathexes. All psychotic patients react to the impact of another person. This sensitivity to external stimuli arising from interpersonal contact was also observed by McGhie and Chapman in the course of their investigations, and details of these reactions are described in Chapter 9. For present purposes it is the nature of these reactions which must be scrutinized. It must be decided whether these universal reactions are identical with the transferences that characterize neurotic patients.

The observable phenomena suggest that the non-specific reactions belong to a level of mental organization which bears similarities to that of the infant of under eight months. At that time objects do not have an independent existence apart from needs, and thus are an indivisible

part of the rudimentary self. In those patients who primarily demonstrate such non-specific reactivity, there is a similar relationship to
objects. Their existence and the attitudes which develop towards them
are entirely based upon needs. In Chapter 10 Cameron describes the
manner in which patients of this type relate during treatment.

When these phenomena are interpreted theoretically it would be
correct to say that, at this 'need-satisfying' level of mental functioning
(A. Freud, 1952), object-libidinal cathexes are in abeyance or lost forever. The reappearance of such a psychic organization implies that the
patient is incapable of transference, which is dependent upon neutralized object-libidinal cathexes. It can be further hypothesized that,
although the diffuse non-specific reactivity is a form of repetition (repetition of early infantile reactions), it is to be distinguished from the
repetitive patterns arising from later developmental phases (self-object
discrimination; object constancy (A. Freud, 1952)) which constitute
the transference manifestations. Transferences are repetitions, but it does
not follow that all repetitive phenomena are transferences. Transference depends upon self-object discrimination and the capacity to invest
objects with neutralized cathexes.

The position adopted here is that there are in fact two separate groups
of reactions. The reactivity that characterizes all psychotic patients
is diffuse and not specific for any one individual. It may be, but is not
necessarily, a repetition phenomenon as in the case of true transferences.
The following is a case in point.

CASE 4. The patient was a man of thirty-six who had been hospitalized
for some years. He was deluded, hallucinated, and presented a severe
degree of disorganization of both thinking and perceiving. The data
to be described occurred against a background of an impending
interruption of a continuous clinical contact which was under way. The
patient had been told about the break.

During this particular interview the patient was characteristically
withdrawn and apathetic. It was impossible to follow the few utterances
he made, on account of the fragmentation of speech and thinking.
Strenuous attempts were made to get him to discuss the fact that there
would be no meetings for about four weeks, but without effect. He
remained silent or smiled for no apparent reason. When the session
ended the interviewer stopped in the ward to talk to an attendant.
Another patient came over to speak, and while this was happening the
patient in question walked over to the little group. He stood listening

for a moment or two then suddenly burst into a fit of rage. He berated the interviewer for coming a few minutes late, which had in fact happened. He screamed out that he had not been on holiday for five years but no one cared. After this, he stamped off and a few hours later he reverted to his withdrawn state.

This patient was sensitive to the interviewer, but it was a sensitivity that was rarely observable. Prior to this outburst he had had a prolonged daily contact with the interviewer and no sign of a specific relationship patterning had occurred. The patient was indifferent to the interviewer, but this indifference could not be compared with that of the non-psychotic patient whose attendance for interviews, if nothing else, reveals his attachment to the therapy. In this case the patient had to be sought out for interviews. At a later stage of the clinical contact this man reacted with depression of mood and later anger when the interviewer could not comply with wishes that were an integral aspect of his delusional complex.

In contrast to this non-specific, diffuse, and sporadic reactivity is the response of those psychotic patients who develop working transferences and whose behaviour in the interview situation soon assumes specific patterns. This development was to be observed in the following case (Case 5). An account will be given here of the first eight weeks of a five-month observation period, during which the patient was seen five times per week.

CASE 5. The patient was a fifty-year-old married woman who had been admitted to mental hospital on one previous occasion some four months prior to the period of observation. During her first stay in hospital, which lasted about four weeks, she stated that she was convinced that she was being followed, watched, and victimized by unknown persons who she imagined were friends of people she had unwittingly antagonized. She was self-reproachful, but could not believe that she deserved the anticipated punishment. She was depressed in mood. She was inclined to misinterpret events so that they could fall in with her delusional ideas. However, there was no sign of hallucinatory phenomena nor any evidence whatever of passivity feelings or of ideas of being controlled.

Treatment by phenothiazines led to a weakening of her irrational ideation, but even at the time of discharge she was not convinced that her experiences had been imaginary. The depressive mood was relieved. When this patient returned to hospital some four months later she was in a state almost identical with that found during her first admission. It was during this stay in hospital that she was interviewed daily for about five months. During this period she was without any form of medication apart from an occasional hypnotic at night.

Material elicited during the eight weeks revealed that the patient's illness appeared about the time that her only child — a son aged twenty-two — decided to leave home, abandoning his occupation for one his mother disapproved of. The relapse occurred about the time when he announced his engagement. The patient's early childhood was very unsettled. She had many changes of house, and when she was seven her father abandoned the family. She lived with different relatives, was sent to an orphanage with her brother, and then lived with an alcoholic grandmother. Her brother went off to the Army when she was about fourteen and she never saw him again. Separations and disappointments seemed to recur constantly throughout her life.

The phenomena that appeared within the context of the patient-observer situation can be best described in two ways. First, an overall picture can be given by describing the predominant attitudes which the patient developed towards the observer and, second, a further account can be conveyed by a week-by-week statement of the proceedings.

The patient related to the observer in a number of different ways. At first she regarded him as an associate of the persecutors. She looked upon him as a kind of examiner and at one time thought he was a policeman. There were other times when she thought of him as an *agent provocateur* who would get her to incriminate herself. At a later time she came to regard him as her principal persecutor. She endowed him with omnipotence and omniscience. She believed he controlled her mind and body and could influence her thinking and bodily processes. Most often she conceived of this power as being associated with the hypnotic state. Within this context she accused the observer of being a sadist, a torturer, and one who was gratified by her suffering. A further attitude was one of curiosity about the examiner, and later there appeared a mixture of negativism and hostility which lasted for almost the whole of the sixth and seventh week of the observation period. This later attitude had a special mental content associated with it. Throughout she insisted that the observer hated her. Finally she demonstrated a dependency and a dread of separation.

The latter phenomena made their initial appearance at the end of the second week and at subsequent weekend breaks. They were also manifested on an occasion when the observer said goodbye after a mid-week session and were equally pronounced after the patient was told of the termination date of the sessions. The patient presented this separation fear at the second and third weekends in the context of a fear of the other patients' jealousy and envy of her previous good health and her husband and son. She felt protected while being seen by the observer but unprotected at the weekends when he was away.

When the patient's material is examined in detail, the first week and a half are characterized by her view of the observer as an agent of the persecutors. On the Friday of week 2, however, she revealed her belief that he was influencing and controlling her. On the Friday of week 2 and on Monday and Tuesday of week 3 she blamed the observer for interfering with her bodily sensibility. She had no appetite, and experienced a wooden feeling inside and a numbness of the skin of the face and limbs. She believed that she would recover sensation later in order to suffer every kind of symptom (usually those which other patients in the ward complained about).

On the Wednesday of week 3 she attacked another patient, saying she was influencing her. The cause of this attack only appeared during week 5. She accused the observer of interfering with her internal organs and while doing so adopted threatening postures – she said, 'I can feel you hating me.' The next day her son came up from England to visit her. Until this time she had been convinced he was dead. His visit led to an improvement in her mental state and to the disappearance of the delusional ideas centring on the observer.

The beneficial change continued for the remainder of week 3. However, she showed considerable separation fear at the weekend in the manner described above. On the Monday of week 4 the 'psychotic transference' returned in full force, but by the Tuesday it was gone. Although convinced of the observer's powers, she no longer felt that her body was under influence. The Wednesday of week 4 brought a return of these 'psychotic transferences'. This return was associated in the patient's mind with the observer saying 'goodbye' after the Tuesday meeting. Thursday and Friday of week 4 found her free of delusional ideas concerning the observer. During this time she related details of her deprived childhood and, of especial importance, the wish that her son would die. This wish had occupied her mind after he had left home.

When the patient was seen on Monday of week 5 she believed once again that the observer controlled her. She called the weekend her 'angry weekend' because of her rage against the observer. She called him 'Satan' for putting bad thoughts in her head. On Tuesday and

Wednesday there was no sign of this material, but on Thursday the 'psychotic transference' had reappeared. She had a letter from her son telling about himself and his fiancée. It is important to note that the patient's illness began at the time when her son left home and recurred when he announced his engagement.

On Friday of week 5 she accused the observer of persecuting her sexually. She said that continuously for the past two weeks he had arranged for sexual interference in the night. She had evidence that she was forced to go out into the grounds and participate in disgusting sexual activities with an older man. She heard other patients reporting this. This had started some days before she attacked the other patient, during week 3. She had done this because this woman was implicated in the persecution. Her belief was based on the fact that she had noted some vaginal bleeding during the second week of the observation period. (The patient's menses had ceased two years previously.) A gynaecological examination carried out later did not reveal any abnormality to account for this vaginal bleeding.

Monday of week 6 brought new revelations. She was hostile and negativistic, a pattern that was to continue for the next ten days. She told the observer that he had made her think Saturday was Friday. She was standing waiting to go to the interview and at that moment he had made her experience sexual sensations. She hated him — he was a torturer and a sadist. After this outburst she revealed that, as a child of eleven, she had been seduced by a grocer for whom she did errands. At this period of her life she had virtually no relationships, for her grandmother, with whom she lived, was a drunkard and her grandfather was away from home. It is unnecessary here to give details of her deprived childhood. She hated the observer from the start because he had reminded her of the grocer. In both cases she felt loathing and disgust yet was unable to keep away.

Concern with sexual persecution only continued for a further two days — by Thursday it had disappeared. A letter from her son accentuated her belief that he was either mentally ill or a drug addict. She believed he was weak-willed. She remained hostile and reluctant to talk. She was convinced of the observer's omnipotence and believed that some substance was being put in her food to keep her under control. She remained in this state until the end of the week.

Week 7 began with a denial of concern about anything. She announced that she had been happy at the weekend with day-dreams, but still believed that she was under a hypnotic influence. She was reluctant to attend the interviews and was mildly unco-operative. This pattern characterized her mental state until the Wednesday when she was told that the daily meetings would be temporarily interrupted in ten days' time. The next day she was angry and tantalized the observer by saying that she had something special in her mind but was not going to reveal what it was. She added that once the meetings stopped she would be changed in such a way that she would be without memory or identity.

In spite of her intention, she eventually revealed that the observer reminded her of her hated father who had abandoned the family when she was about seven years old. This equation of father and observer explained some of the patient's earlier curiosity about the latter. For some days during the early weeks she had been preoccupied with the observer's height, the size of shoes he wore, and other physical characteristics.

On the Friday of week 7 she once again began to complain about alteration in bodily sensibility. The hostility and negativism which had been present disappeared. She complained that her memory was slowly being obliterated and that a numbness was spreading over her body. She felt empty inside and without feeling apart from sadness. This was all the observer's doing. By Monday of week 8 there was a change in the content of the delusions. She no longer complained of persecution, thinking instead that the removal of her memory and identity would protect her from painful news of her son's death in disgrace. However, for the remainder of the week persecutory ideas returned with varying degrees of overt hostility towards the observer. She continued to complain of the change in bodily sensations and the imminent loss of memory and identity. She freely expressed her concern that she would no longer see the observer and was frightened that something might happen to him.

During the next four weeks (weeks 9–13) there was a revival of persecutory ideas regarding the investigator and these were associated with negativism and hostility. The patient did not want to attend the meetings. However, after the difficult week she revealed a short-lived spell of infidelity to her husband about a year or so before the outbreak of the symptoms. It was impossible to ignore the obvious sexualization of the interview situation and the patient freely admitted – without prompting – her equation of clinician and lover. This revelation was followed by a suicidal attempt which came to nothing. Finally, she revealed another traumatic experience which further explained her persecutory delusions and intense guilt feelings.

In this case psychotic phenomena displaced to the interviewer (psychotic transferences) appeared side by side with genuine transference manifestations. The patient made the strongest attachment to the investigator and from the beginning transferred her phantasies about her father, her childhood seducer, and her lover onto him. These phantasies provoked intense transference resistance until they were able to attain verbalization. She displaced the annoyance and discontent she felt about her husband onto the interviewer but at different times. The psychotic manifestations that appeared were the persecutory ideas and the attributing to the investigator of a magical omnipotence (projection of psychotic narcissism).

The return of the repressed that made itself manifest in the transference neurosis followed an orderly sequence, thus reflecting the organized nature of the repressed contents. Phenomena relating to the physician that find expression in more severe forms of psychosis than the present case suggest that what has been repressed is completely disorganized, as is the remainder of mental and physical functioning. Lack of organization within the repressed reflects the cathectic disturbance that has affected the endopsychic object relationships. It follows from this that an analytic situation could not, in any circumstances, lead to anything other than the transfer of isolated, disconnected, and disorganized contents. A transference neurosis of the kind observable in the above-mentioned case is therefore absent in these severely disturbed patients. All that can be discerned is a non-specific reactivity the latent meaning of which can only be surmised. It may be possible, as Searles (1963a) maintains and as Cameron describes in Chapter 10, to put together those isolated fragments and note the presence of something akin to a transference neurosis after many years of treatment.

PSYCHO-ANALYTIC RECORDING IN PSYCHOSIS

The essence of the technique involved in the psycho-analytic observation of psychotic patients consists in the observer's confining his interpretative communications to the analysis of unconscious resistances. The content should be limited as far as possible to the patient's utterances and behaviour in the consulting-room and how they relate to himself. In favourable circumstances the patient may bring historical material which will give meaning to the behaviour. By limiting himself to communications of this type, the investigator is in less danger of contaminating the field than would be the case if he were to make interpretations of unconscious content, which must in the nature of things be highly inferential and many stages removed from the clinical data. This technique offers the observer a means of noting the development of both neurotic and 'psychotic' transferences. It also gives him the opportunity of discovering the principal defensive measures (resistances) employed by the patient's ego organization.

Throughout this discussion, emphasis has been laid upon the importance of what occurs within the clinical setting because of its potential for yielding information about the state of the patient's interpersonal relationships. This information must be recorded in order that it can be examined with regard to its connections with the symptomatology and cognitive functioning. Thus the psychotic patient's initial reactions to the observer's situation must be gauged in just the same way as with the psychoneurotic reaction. A preliminary estimate of the patient's capacity to enter into the relationship must be made because this will give an approximate idea of the extent of the psychotic involvement. This must be followed by an assessment of the patient's behaviour and attitude in the observation situation. Note will be made as to whether the patient is respectful, dependent, fearful, impatient, curious, concerned about the observer's welfare, afraid of criticism, sexually interested, or afraid of harming the observer.

The study of psychoneurotic reactions by means of the psycho-analytic method has shown repeatedly that, at the outset, patients are afraid to reveal their conscious and pre-conscious thoughts and feelings about the treatment and the psycho-analyst. Nevertheless, their hidden attitudes reveal themselves in the course of their free associations. Among the commonest allusions to the analyst are remarks about other doctors, teachers, parents, or spouses. When the patient is confronted with his fear of expressing these hidden thoughts, he usually admits them with relief and with a resultant gain in confidence in the analyst.

The clinician must always be on the lookout for allusions to hidden resentment, hostility, sexual interest, and all the other attitudes which have been described. For example, a young female psychotic patient who showed the greatest reluctance to discuss her difficulties was talking about a visit to her mother and said that she was very angry when her mother's lover had burst into her room while she was dressing. At a later interview she recalled that a reporter had pestered her for information while she was working in a hospital. Both these statements were allusions to her distaste for the treatment and her disinclination to talk. She regarded the physician as an intruder. In order to reduce the possibility of the observer's reading incorrect meaning into the patient's utterances and behaviour, it is important for him to refrain from coming to hard-and-fast conclusions about the meaning of a particular piece of content until the patient has produced confirmation of it.

Unlike the psychoneurotic patient, the psychotic patient will show those additional reactions, so-called 'psychotic' transferences, to which reference has already been made and which are characteristic of his mental state. Deficiencies in perceptual function may lead him to confuse himself with the observer and with others in his immediate environment. This was the case with the female patient who came into the consulting-room, sat down, and began to cough spasmodically and hold her throat. After being questioned about this rather startling behaviour she said that it had occurred when she noticed the observer coughing. Of equal importance is the patient's tendency to confuse the observer with individuals who have had a significance for him.

Resistances will appear during the contact with the psychotic patient in just the same way as they will occur during the psycho-analytic therapy of the neurotic disorder. Those who have had extensive psycho-therapeutic experience with psychotic patients emphasize the intensity and special features of these resistances (see Chapter 10). Negativism, and delusional ideas with persecutory content linked to the observer or therapist, are examples of these resistances. Much of the resistance will be similar to that encountered in the neuroses and will derive from the non-psychotic residues, as in the cases recently described. Clinical experiences suggest that, as in the neuroses, these responses spring from anxiety within the patient. These resistances or defences must also be recorded and assessed because of their close relationship to the symptomatology. It is well known that denial, projection, and reversal play an important part in the creation of delusional content. These mechanisms enable the patient to forgo the repression of unacceptable ideas. The patient can allow such content to enter consciousness because it is ascribed to someone else. In this respect psychotic manifestations differ entirely from psychoneurotic symptoms, where the main purpose of defence is the concealment of the repressed from consciousness.

The patient may similarly utilize introjective mechanisms in order to dissipate hatred of the observer, thus leading to depression, self-criticism, and sometimes to suicidal attempts. This was particularly clear in the case of the middle-aged woman who, after revealing some of her 'secrets' — themselves a declaration of her libidinal phantasies about the therapist — introjected her hatred, which had been awakened by the frustration of these libidinal wishes. Similarly, introjection of the object (the observer) may occur in order to nullify ambivalence or as a reaction to separation. All these possibilities must be considered and allowance made for the sexualization of the observation situation. Once again, the case described above is an excellent example of this, and illustrates how patients' behaviour in the clinical situation is determined by such sexualization. In this case, as in the majority of such instances, there is no overt manifestation of sexuality, but rather a reaction which takes the form of negativism, antagonism, and a tendency to seek sexual outlets outside the observer situation.

A record of projective mechanisms can be made by constructing a series of statements which include the instinctual drive against which the defence is directed. Note must be made of the following: (*a*) unreasonable accusations of the observer being critical of the patient (here an attempt is made to record the projection of conscience — superego); (*b*) complaints that the observer expects too much from the patient (projection of oral demands); (*c*) complaints that the observer wants to find out things about him (projection of scopophilic tendencies); (*d*) assertions that the observer has a sexual (genital) interest in him (projection of homo- or heterosexual drives); (*e*) assertions that the observer is keeping back information from him (projection of anal-retentive tendencies); (*f*) assertions that the observer dislikes him (projection of hostile wishes).

The introjection of aggressive drives can be identified by paying special attention to the presence of depression of mood, feelings of hopelessness, and self-criticism. The introjection of the object is more difficult to assess in psychotic states because it is difficult to differentiate from the fusion of self and object that is so often due to faulty perceptual discrimination.

Further information about resistances and defensive processes can be obtained from the patient's reactions to the observer's communications. The hypothesis of sexualization of the observer's situation to which reference was made above enables a further series of questions to be formulated. They concern: silence as a reaction to the observer's communication, negativistic attitudes, impatience, continual disagreement, and hostility. These phenomena were particularly marked in the case described above. It would be erroneous to assume as, was mentioned earlier, that silence or negativism can only be motivated by

unconscious sexualization of the observer situation, that is, by a transference resistance. The question does however allow the observer the
opportunity to record a specific pattern of patient behaviour whose
cause may indeed lie in unconscious sexualization. Finally, such reactions as disappointment, indifference, anxiety, and compliance with
the observer's comments must also be noted when present.

As the observer or therapist never remains indifferent to his patient
it is important to have some rough check on his conscious reactions.
This record of the observer's reactions is to be distinguished from what
is described as countertransference. The latter is an unconscious
attitude on the part of the therapist towards the patient. Countertransference is difficult to record because its presence can only be inferred.
But with regard to the observer's conscious reaction to the patient
(counter-reaction), the following require to be noted: impatience,
irritation, fear, disgust, anger, neutral feelings, and boredom. It is quite
possible for each topic referred to in the above paragraphs to be detailed in a rating scale which can be assessed at each observation session.
In this way data are obtained daily about the patient-observer situation,
as well as information regarding changes in cognition, affectivity, and
other symptom complexes.

Psycho-analytic theory is employed because it enables the investigator to construct a series of questions which he can try to
answer on the basis of the patient's behaviour and utterances. Further,
psycho-analytic hypotheses suggest that changes will occùr both in the
patient-observer situation and in the symptomatology once specific
mental stresses have been activated. It is conceivable that certain
patients will be vulnerable to separation both at weekends and at holidays
(see Chapter 10). Some of them may react to this stress with hatred
against the observer. This hatred may become conscious or, as a result
of introjection, projection, or repression, it may never achieve this
state. Introjective defences will lead to self-criticism and depression of
mood. The buried hate may lead to the patient becoming fearful for the
observer's welfare or worrying that somehow he may harm him unwittingly. Such reactions may occur just before or immediately after
interruption in the observer relationship.

Psycho-analytic theory also points to the possibility that jealousy and
envy can lead to alteration within the observer-patient situation and to
changes in cognition and other symptoms. Similarly, the dread of
sexual wishes towards an object may have the same effect. A daily
record of the patient's reactions may pinpoint these associations.

Individual studies of this kind can be carried out for any length of time. The employment of psycho-analysis as a research technique for the study of the psychoses widens the field of investigation. Psycho-analytic hypotheses direct the investigator's attention to the unconscious aspects of interpersonal relations and permit an assessment of them in the manner described.

CHAPTER 4

Disturbances of Attention and Concentration

Psycho-analytic theory proposes that in schizophrenic states and allied conditions the capacity to attend is limited on account of certain alterations that affect the ego organization. The theory lays stress on the idea that anxiety arising from the emergence of specific instinctual trends causes a regression within the ego. This regression has a number of effects, among which disintegration of repression and the counter-cathectic barriers is the most important in this particular context. A regression also affects the instinctual basis of object relations, leading to a pathological egocentrism and to the omnipotence of thoughts (psychotic narcissism). The reality of things is replaced by the reality of ideas.

Under normal conditions the counter-cathectic barriers insulate the cognitive functions necessary for environmental adaptation. External stimuli are screened and only those percepts of adaptive value are permitted admission to consciousness. The remainder may achieve mental registration (Klein, 1959) but never reach awareness. An inner counter-cathexis walls off the ego from the special form of activity that characterizes unconscious mental processes — the primary process. This counter-cathexis also ensures the exclusion from consciousness of instinct-ridden ideational contents.

CLINICAL OBSERVATIONS

The psycho-analytic literature on psychotic states is replete with the clinical material upon which this hypothesis rests. These clinical data assume different forms but in each instance they are associated with disturbances in the sphere of interpersonal relations. Two distinct classes of clinical phenomena are relevant here. In the first category the disturbance in interpersonal relations is associated with an inability to achieve freedom from auditory and visual perceptual experience. In such patients there is a loss of the screening function which protects consciousness from external stimulation. Complaints are made that television, wireless, radio waves, or invisible 'rays' are constantly assaulting the patient's mind or body. These may be accompanied by the further complaint that he is unable clearly to discriminate himself as an entity from others or from what he sees on the television screen. In other instances the patient is overwhelmed by a continuous stream of remarks made by others in his immediate vicinity. This bombardment may reach such an intensity that he will plug his ears with cotton-wool. These patients must be distinguished from those who are constantly assailed by hallucinatory voices when they are alone.

Psycho-analysts would suggest that the patient who complained of other people speaking about him in his presence had reached this state because of the breakdown of the internal counter-cathectic barrier. They would say that the affectively toned ideational material which had broken through into the ego had generated anxiety of such an order that it was now projected, so leading to the misinterpretation of such speech as was overheard. The content of these misperceptions would consist of a mixture of the repudiated instinctual needs and the condemnation which the patient made of them. The inner flood is dammed by locating it in the environment, where some control may be achieved by isolation or blocking of perception. Similarly, in hallucinatory states projection distances the patient from the inner source of stimulation (Havens, 1962).

Psychological studies (Frenkel-Brunswik, 1951) have advanced support for the theory that anxiety can lead to a non-veridical concept of reality. In order to obtain release from anxiety or other form of undifferentiated psychic stress, there can be a premature tendency on the part of the individual to come to general conclusions based upon evidence that does not correspond with the actual environmental situation. This process can be thought of as a perversion of a mechanism of 'inductive belief' (Miller, 1951) which normally has the function of enabling the organism to prepare itself for an emergency on the basis of minimal information. In the clinical material to which reference was made above, the anxiety and the misinterpretations (non-veridical concept of reality) excited by it force the patient to avoid further perceptual stimulation.

The second category of clinical data consists of patients with delusions

F

whose content may include grandiose, persecutory, or depressive ideas. This content is derived from memory traces of childhood (Niederland, 1959; Freud, 1937) and from phantasies of various kinds which ordinarily never enter consciousness. These phantasies either express instinctual needs (oral, anal, scoptophilic, sadistic) or represent the patient's dread of retribution on account of such wishes. The supremacy of psychic reality reveals these phantasies to the patient as actual and fulfilled.

The appearance of these forms of psychic content (distorted memory traces, phantasies) in consciousness now in the shape of delusions suggests that a major disruption has affected the internal counter-cathectic barrier. Just as the former group of patients are unable to disengage themselves from external perceptual stimulation so are the latter unable to free themselves from preoccupation with their delusional ideation. In both categories attention is consumed by the flood of stimulation – externalized in one group, internal in the other. Cases who show both kinds of phenomenon are also encountered.

The capacity to attend to a conversation or to a purposive task is seriously affected by those states of mental and physical overactivity which are generally diagnosed as mania or hypomania. In these cases it is often possible to demonstrate that the environmental stimulus which is selected is not chosen at random but is picked because it is associatively linked with an inner preoccupation. A defective counter-cathectic barrier can be evoked to explain this type of clinical phenomenon also.

Failure to sustain attention because of distractability is also found in schizophrenic states. McGhie and Chapman have confirmed this experimentally (see Chapter 9). In such conditions the mental hyperactivity regarded as typical of manic states may be absent. The distractability that occurs in these cases of schizophrenia is most commonly found in the hebephrenic form of the illness – a finding again confirmed by McGhie and Chapman in Chapter 9. It has been observed that the inverse relationship which appears to exist between the capacity to attend and the degree of distractability will fluctuate in accordance with the extent of the hebephrenic deterioration. As the cognitive dysfunction which characterizes the hebephrenic process diminishes, the distractability lessens and the patient's capacity for sustained attention improves. This sequence of events has been seen in association with changes in interpersonal relationships and during drug therapy. It is equally possible for these changes to occur in the reverse order – the disappearance of delusions being followed by cognitive dysfunction, distractability, and an inability to sustain attention.

A PSYCHO-ANALYTIC THEORY OF ATTENTION

Under normal conditions the individual can freely give his attention to the environment or to his thoughts. He is equally able to disengage his attention if it becomes necessary to focus it upon a matter of greater urgency. Attention must therefore be freely mobile and yet capable of being rapidly concentrated upon a specific pattern of perceptual experience, either of thought or of the environment. Without this ability the individual is hampered in his capacity for optimal adaptation. According to psycho-analytic theory, a deterioration in the function of attention is initiated by specific endopsychic stresses, which are in turn activated by environmental circumstances. Psycho-analytic theory, however, does not confine itself to this one approach. It also emphasizes the need to understand the nature of the attentive process itself.

In his original conception of mental function (mental apparatus concept), Freud (1900) regarded consciousness as a sense organ which was in receipt of stimuli from both the environment and the interior. This concept, in contrast to his later formulations on this topic, is of great value in trying to come to an understanding of the abnormalities which may affect purposive attention. Freud (1900) believed that percepts arising in the environment did not make an instantaneous appearance in consciousness but first passed through an unconscious phase. Experimental psychologists have advanced evidence in favour of such a theory of perception. They suggest that there are stages of the perceptual process during which the memory traces of visual stimuli, for example, pass through a series of transformations before they become conscious as images or visual percepts. A distinction is drawn (Klein, 1959) between the registration of perceptual data — occurring unconsciously — and consciousness of percepts. 'Unconscious' in this context need not imply the presence of associated repressed contents and defences like denial (see Chapter 2). The perceptual data in their first phases are not necessarily unconscious because of anxiety (unconscious in the dynamic sense) but may be, as Schilder (1923) pointed out, organically unconscious. This distinction has more than academic interest because there are schizophrenic patients who deny awareness of an environmental percept while at the same time betraying through their utterances that it has achieved registration outside consciousness. In such a case a decision must be made as to whether this inattention is psychologically motivated or whether the disease process has led to a defect of the attention mechanism itself.

Fundamental to the psycho-analytic theory of consciousness is the idea of attention being an active process. While it may be passively activated by external stimulation or by the vivid imagery of the dream, adaptation to the world necessitates a function which is constantly searching out and locating, for subsequent examination, data in the immediate environment and in the inner milieu of verbal and memory schemata. Preconscious mental contents can only become conscious when they are invested with a special quantity of cathectic energy – a hypercathexis. Attention, which is purposive in aim, is synonymous with the distribution of additional cathexes directed to selected ideational contents or to specific external events. Conceptual thinking, in terms of this hypothesis, is therefore dependent upon an active mental process initiated by the sense organ of consciousness.

The psycho-analytic study of dreams offers the observer a view of the attentive process which is not accessible in acts of sustained concentration. This aspect of attention is similar in many respects to the role which it often assumes in psychotic states. In the dream attention passively turns to those dream images which possess the greatest sensory intensity. This intensity results from the condensation of numerous ideas which are associatively linked. Displacement ensures that an inverse relationship exists between the psychical significance of a dream image and its sensory intensity.

The dreamer's attention is captured and held fast by dream images in just the same manner as psychotic patients are unable to banish from awareness the perceptual bombardment arising from the environment or from thought. Examples of this type of clinical data were referred to above. The patient is unable to direct his attention purposively because it is so completely enmeshed by perceptual experience. Rapaport (1951) is referring to this kind of clinical data when he says that hallucinations, delusions, and other psychotic phenomena are not dependent upon a hypercathectic process for entry into consciousness as is the case with purposive thinking. Their appearance is automatic because they are not primarily sought out by consciousness. They attract and imprison attention. The attentive process has assumed a passive role in such states, which is to be contrasted with its activity in the performance of sustained and directed concentration.

FURTHER CLINICAL DATA

It is now time to turn once again to the disturbances of attention that occur in psychotic states. As in the previous discussion, the concepts to be employed are drawn from psycho-analytic theory. This does not imply that other conceptualizations — psychological or neurophysiological (Lindsley, 1960) — are less valuable or that they are unable to offer a comprehensive explanation of the phenomena. The psycho-analytic approach is preferred because, in the words of Adrian (1946), psycho-analytic concepts are closer to the observed data than, for example, are neurophysiological constructs. This approximation affords the investigator a method of ordering the clinical material in terms of the patient's current state, his life experiences, and the psychical reactions they engendered. At the same time, no one can doubt that these psychological events, however conceptualized, which have their own reality, must in the end be extrapolations from neurophysiological function.

When patients suffering from functional psychoses are exposed to close examination it would seem that an obvious disorder of attention is not a universal occurrence. There are many patients, particularly those who fall into the categories of the paranoid state and paranoid schizophrenia, who appear to be able to attend adequately to a set task or to join in a conversation. This observation was also made by Chapman and McGhie in their experimental studies (see Chapter 9). Concentration does not seem to be impaired in any way. Observations of this type, however, cannot be taken at face value. An analogy might be drawn with disordered physiological functions which give a normal response, as evidenced by some objective criterion, while the activity is not subjected to stress. Once a demand is made upon the particular function the response is clearly abnormal. It may be, therefore, that in paranoid states there is only a semblance of an adequately functioning attentive process. The application of stress may reveal an underlying abnormality.

Distractability by external stimuli is the clinical phenomenon which best reflects a defect in the capacity to attend and concentrate on a given task. Reference has already been made to the possibility that this distraction from without represents a means of dealing with an internal stress from which there is no escape. A woman patient's fear of her husband's infidelity, for example, was reflected in her attention being constantly deflected from the discussion in hand to the floral design of the carpet. Flora, Rose, Blossom, Violet, and other names of this kind continually preoccupied the patient's mind because they were identical with or similar to the names of young women who were employed by her husband. Only through questioning did the patient's fear become manifest and simultaneously provided the explanation for the content of the distracting percepts.

Distractability has been explained as resulting from a deficiency in the capacity to selectively attend. This selectivity is dependent upon the ability to isolate thoughts or percepts from the remainder of mental activity and environmental stimuli. As was seen above, the concept of counter-cathexis is employed in psycho-analytic theory to explain this function. Neurophysiological theories of attention call upon the concept of inhibition — emphasizing the role of the mid-brain reticular formation in reducing sensory input to uninvolved areas of the cortex (Gellhorn & Loofbourrow, 1963). Distractability is not confined to the overactive patient, but, as mentioned above, is to be found in the apathetic, withdrawn, cognitively deteriorated patient of hebephrenic type. As with the manic patient, it is often possible to discern the motivation behind the perception of the distracting stimulus.

When the distractability of the manic or hypomanic patient is scrutinized it becomes apparent that he is constantly scanning the environment for sources of stimulation. It is the rapid movement of attention from one subject to the next that constitutes the distractability. As in the case of the hypomanic woman and her flower names, the perceptual data are often selected in accordance with orectic factors. In mania and hypomania, attention is not passively attracted to objects but is actively directed to them. This stands in contrast to schizophrenic and paranoid patients whose attention is passively tied to hallucinatory experiences or to falsified perceptions.

In those occasional instances when a chronic hebephrenic patient becomes distracted, the clinician can observe in slow motion the sequence of events that occurs so rapidly in mania. This may lead to a break in the patient's communications and to the inappropriate appearance of a new theme. A young hebephrenic man was asking whether he could have a scar removed by plastic surgery. While he was talking a man called Gunn entered the room. Immediately following this and without any alteration in his manner of speech, he introduced some remarks about Stevenson's novel *Treasure Island* and the character Ben Gunn. This led him to the name Robinson and to complaints about fellow-patients whom he regarded as dangerous.

It is not inconceivable that the connection between Ben Gunn and Robinson is Robinson Crusoe who was also marooned on a desert island. It may be that the name Gunn was a means whereby the patient could express – in a condensed and symbolic form – his own plight. He was also marooned and surrounded by unpredictable and aggressive 'savages'. In contrast to the manic patient the attentive process in cases such as the one described is not characterized by hyperactivity. It is essentially passive and only occasionally caught up by sense impressions which are associatively connected with an inner preoccupation.

Clinical phenomena of this type, combined with the knowledge that in chronic hebephrenia there is a tendency to assimilate fragments of overheard speech and observed behaviour (Freeman, Cameron & McGhie, 1958) have been partly instrumental in leading to the theory that in schizophrenia the individual has lost the ability to insulate consciousness from environmental stimulation. Some support has been found for this theory by psychologists engaged on the study of perceptual processes. Klein (1959) has suggested that registration of external stimuli within the healthy mind occurs on a wider and more indiscriminate scale than could ever have been imagined on the basis of observable reactions. This writer puts forward the idea that there are 'controlling structures' which govern the fate of these mental registrations. They remain unconscious or find their way into consciousness as percepts or images.

In cases of chronic hebephrenia the observer may note a situation not unlike that which Klein (1959) conceives as occurring unconsciously in the healthy individual. The patient frequently makes it clear that he is the recipient of a flood of stimuli. Registration and perception are no longer separate activities but seem to run into one another. This clinical impression finds support in Poetzl's assertion that in psychotic states patients become aware of percepts which ordinarily remain unconscious. It is possible to envisage a mental state in chronic hebephrenia where what remains of the ego is at once overcome by the demands of the instincts and by a barrage of environmental stimuli which reach consciousness as percepts or images to the detriment of reality adaptation.

The failure to utilize the function of attention in schizophrenic and allied states can be observed in yet another sphere. A passing reference was made to this phenomenon of perceptual inattention. The deficiency can be seen in both early and late cases. In chronic hebephrenia it is often impossible to get the patient to respond to external stimulation. This stimulation may be auditory, as in the case of con-versation, or visual. It appears as if the stimulus has failed to make any impact. The patient remains silent, continues with his own utter-ances, or responds with motor behaviour. A clinical example may illustrate this more clearly. A patient was given a box of chocolates for his birthday. The chocolates were manufactured by a company named Duncan. The patient ignored the gift throughout the interview, talking in his own peculiar fragmented way about his artistic talents. On a number of occasions he referred to a man called Duncan, sug-gesting that the gift had registered in his mind. In Klein's (1959) terminology, awareness of the percept did not occur because attention was not actively deployed to the mental registration of what had been presented to perception. In this example attention failed to respond to a specific stimulus not because of a failure to inhibit extraneous stimula-tion but because other mental contents held a greater attraction for it. Attention was thus characterized by a passivity quite opposite to that necessary for sustained concentration. It had been reduced to a process of passive assimilation.

Reference was made earlier to the fact that attention is not obviously disturbed in the majority of paranoid disorders. An opportunity was afforded of witnessing such a disturbance in a patient who would other-wise have been thought normal in this particular respect. The fifty-year-old woman patient referred to in Chapter 3 suffered from persecutory delusions without any defect of thought or perceptual processes. She was submitted to a test which consisted of her having to press a key in response to the appearance of a light. A little later she had to press the key again while exposed simultaneously to the visual and a new audi-tory stimulus. The apparatus had two lights, one red and one blue, and two keys for the right and left hands. The lights were flashed in different sequences.

From the start of the test the patient was completely fixated to the key corresponding to the red light. She could not transfer her attention to the blue light when it flashed. This tendency was accentuated by the introduction of the auditory stimulus. The explanation of this fail-ure to attend was presented by the patient spontaneously at a clinical interview held the next day. She had become distressed immediately she had perceived the red light. Red meant danger, and it was impos-sible for her to withdraw her attention from it and from the associations it awakened. Thoughts about her husband and son, sexual anxieties, and traumatic scenes of childhood prevented her from attending to the blue light and operating the key (see Chapters 3 and 7). All these thoughts had a place in her delusional ideas. Under stress — admittedly accidental in this case — this patient's attention lost its active, autonomous character. The deficiency in the attentive process in this case can be likened to that encountered in the chronic hebephrenic patient who was unable to concentrate upon visual or auditory stimuli. He was preoccupied with his own ideas.

THEORETICAL CONSIDERATIONS

In order to simplify further discussion, only the defects of attention that occur in the schizophrenias and paranoid states will be considered. The hypothesis is advanced here that in the schizophrenias and allied conditions attentive disturbances fall into two extreme forms. In the one case purposive attention fails because the individual is unable to insulate awareness from perceptual stimulation. Percepts on different levels of organizational complexity interfere with the attention mechanism and thus distract him from his current undertaking. In the second group are the patients who cannot concentrate upon a particular stimulus because attention has become fixed to other mental contents.

In the first category attention has lost its active, mobile quality. A train of thought is interrupted by external stimuli other than those appropriate for the continuation of the theme. Motor responses may not be confined to speech but may also consist of bodily movements. In one case of chronic hebephrenia continued conversation with the patient was impossible because his attention was diverted by the sound of a car or an aeroplane or an auditory hallucination. Preoccupation with these stimuli was accompanied by a simultaneous tapping of the foot, vertical movements of the trunk, tapping the head, or making writing movements on his sleeve.

In the second category the patient is wholly preoccupied with specific mental contents. In such a case attention is impossible because the attentive capacity is taken up by hallucinations or delusional experiences. A case in point was that of a married woman of forty-two years whose sole complaint was of voices which appeared to have the function of confusing her regarding her identity, her moral standards, and her life circumstances. She could not work or attend to her household tasks. Attention was passively directed to these hallucinations.

When the two categories are compared it would appear that in the former group extraneous stimuli are assimilated indiscriminately.

There is often an accompanying breakdown of the mechanisms which protect motor functions from sensory stimulation, as in the case quoted above. There is some evidence to favour the theory that such phenomena represent the intrusion of a form of mental activity similar in nature to that obtaining during a phase of infantile development. This undifferentiated and unorganized level of mental development has been described as sensori-motor by genetic psychologists (Piaget, 1947; Werner, 1948), partly because of the lack of inhibitory influences upon perception and motility when the individual is subjected to sensory stimulation. It is of interest that disorganization of the visual capacity (loss of shape, size, and distance constancy) is most often found in patients whose attentive defect is of the first kind. In the second category of attention defect there is no evidence of such sensori-motor activity. This suggests that these patients, in contrast to the others, have not suffered such a serious degree of mental disorganization. These theoretical considerations arising from clinical observations suggest therefore that there are indeed two separate forms of attention defect in the schizophrenias and paranoid psychoses.

There is a possibility that the differentiation of two categories of attention defect is artificial and arbitrary. It could be said that they are merely aspects of a unitary process. In the one case the difficulty arises from excessive, ill-integrated external stimulation, whereas in the other it is a matter of distraction from within. The psycho-analytic approach would, at first sight, tend to support this unitary conception. Reference has been made on more than one occasion to those patients who so misinterpret and falsify their auditory percepts that they believe everything they hear refers to themselves. Such patients cannot sustain attention. The psycho-analytic view mentioned before emphasizes the idea that the dread of auditory perception which appears in these patients reflects the terror of inner dangers which can only be avoided by projection. It is a basic psycho-analytic tenet that ideational contents which give rise to mental pain are located outside the self during the early stages of mental development. This pattern becomes the prototype for the method of dealing with what is unpleasurable. Only with the appearance of the reality principle is this projection tendency limited in its application. It is also true that the psychoanalyst will tend to regard distracting stimuli as determined by preconscious or unconscious interests.

In spite of the support which psycho-analytic theory correctly advances, there are certain considerations to suggest that the aforementioned hypothesis may have some foundation in fact and that distractibility and preoccupation are not merely facets of a unitary process. The failure to sustain attention in the class of patient characterized by falsified auditory perception is not due to distractability by external stimuli. In these cases, as psycho-analysis shows, it is a preoccupation with projected psychic contents to which attention is passively turned. These cases must be categorized with the delusional states and with those others who are refractory to perceptual stimuli. This group must be contrasted with those schizophrenic patients whose communications show that they are indeed distracted because of a failure to insulate thinking and motor behaviour from extraneous stimulation. In these cases attention is not merely reduced to a passive assimilatory process but may be actually disorganized because of the breakdown of counter-cathexes (inhibitory influences) and faulty perceptual discrimination. The results which McGhie & Chapman have obtained in their experimental studies support this view, in so far as it is hebephrenic rather than the paranoid patients who show the greatest impairment of selective attention when asked to perform simple tasks under distracting conditions (see Chapter 9). It is hypothesized, therefore, that a qualitative difference exists between the two forms of defective purposive attention. In one instance attention is disorganized; in the other the capacity for sustained attention is replaced by a passive assimilatory condition similar to that encountered in the dream. The latter statement merely rephrases Rapaport's (1951) assertion that, while purposive attention is characterized by a hypercathexis of thought, delusions and hallucinations find their way into consciousness automatically without such a hypercathexis. It may be that it is only in those schizophrenic states (hebephrenias) characterized by serious cognitive dysfunction that attention becomes disorganized.

It was the observation that cognitive activities fluctuated in their level of efficiency which led Bleuler (1911) to propose that disturbances of concentration, perception, and memory were not primary symptoms. The disturbances of purposive attention which have been described are not static phenomena. Alterations in this function are constantly taking place and the patient who has great difficulty in concentrating one day may be able to attend the next. Similarly, the characteristics of the attention defect may alter, so that on some occasions distractability may be a prominent manifestation while at another time it is replaced by an unresponsiveness or by a concentration on topics other than those immediately relevant. These changes are best exemplified by references to clinical data.

CASE 6. The case in question is a man of forty-six who had suffered from hebephrenic illness for many years. The condition was characterized by an alternation between states of mental and physical hyperactivity, on the one hand, and retardation, apathy, and dullness, on the other. During the hyperactive phases thinking, as reflected in his verbalizations, was under pressure, fragmented, and difficult to follow because of incoherence. Faulty perceptual discrimination found expression in misidentifications and a difficulty in differentiating the self from others in his immediate circle. The hyperactivity was usually accompanied by grandiose and persecutory delusions which were fleeting, fragmented, and in no way systematized. The capacity to sustain attention with regard to either his own thoughts or the environment was poor. Distractability was a commonplace while he was in this state.

When the patient passed into a 'dull' phase his thinking showed signs of retardation, the fragmentation became less marked, and there was less difficulty in following his communications, although the content (delusions) was no less disordered. Perceptual upsets became less pronounced and the capacity to concentrate improved. Concomitantly he became self-critical, with delusional self-reproach and depression in mood. The change from the overactive to the dull phase occurred gradually and even in the latter state there were still signs of cognitive dysfunction.

A short sequence of material may be presented to illustrate the changes which may affect the attentive capacity. This period began when the patient was hyperactive. Outstanding was his inability to preserve the autonomy of his body scheme and his individuality. He would assume the behaviour of the observer and express ideas and beliefs which he, often correctly, believed were characteristic of him. At the same time he attributed to the latter his own bodily sensations and feelings. His ability to concentrate on a question or discussion was limited. He could not sustain a theme because of being easily distracted by a word which had another significance for him. Similarly he tended to incorporate visual and auditory percepts into his utterances.

The inability to attend actively in the overactive phase revealed all the different forms of disturbance described above. At times this patient showed the scanning character which attention takes in manic states. On other occasions his attention was completely disorganized — percepts of different kinds being interspersed between utterances to be followed by non-adaptive behaviour. Simultaneously, his attention would be attracted by a word of significance and this would lead to a delusional fragment. He would frequently ignore the observer's questions because his attention was fixed to mental contents which were important to him. Finally, his capacity to concentrate was seriously impeded by his inability to separate himself off as an entity from the objects of his environment with which he seemed to be fused.

Much of this discussion has been devoted to a clinical description of the disturbances of purposive attention and concentration which occur in the functional psychoses. As far as schizophrenic states are concerned, it is hypothesized that the attentive difficulty falls into two categories: in one, attention assumes a passive assimilatory form and, in the other, there seems to be a disorganization of the attentive process itself running parallel to the general mental disintegration. The former abnormality tends to occur in cases where delusional ideas are well formed, while the latter defect is most often found in cases of hebephrenia, in which there is fairly clear evidence of an extensive disorganization of thought and perceptual activity.

PURPOSIVE ATTENTION AS AN INDEX OF COGNITIVE FUNCTIONING

The capacity to sustain attention requires a maximal integration of optimally functioning cognitive processes. The ability to attend and concentrate could be thought of as a measure of the normality of cognition because it appears at first sight to be dependent upon intact thought and perceptual processes. Thus far, references to the potential for sustained attention have been confined to that aspect of the cognitive organization concerned with the exclusion of stimuli which might have a disrupting effect. Thinking is a central activity of the cognitive organization which serves purposive attention. Thoughts find conscious representation through the agency of verbal symbols. Words provide a framework for conceptual thinking and thus distinguish it from the primitive conceptualizations which characterize the thought processes of the dreamer, the young child, or those from less developed cultures. There exists in the healthy a hierarchy of concepts which is organized according to the degree of abstraction inherent in the concept.

Rapaport (1951) has clarified Schilder's original inquiries into the pathology of conceptual thinking. He has pointed out that concepts have an autonomy once they have achieved their maximal development. Words representing things and ideas come to enjoy, in the course of task- and problem-solving, a freedom from intrusion by other ideas with which they may have been associatively or symbolically linked during early phases of development. Thus concepts enable the individual to perceive and order the world in a meaningful way and, with this as a basis, to contemplate and initiate appropriate behaviour. It is the presence of concepts — discrete and autonomous verbal ideas — which enabled Freud (1900) to describe purposive thinking as a form of trial action. Purposive attending cannot therefore be treated in isolation from the other cognitive functions of which it is a part.

This applies equally to perceptual processes and particularly to the visual modality. Hilgard (1951) proposes that the goals of perception are twofold. First is the creation of environmental stability. In order to achieve this, visual percepts must be characterized by constancies of various kinds. Both objects and the environment must remain relatively consistent with regard to the manner in which they present themselves to perception. The second aim of the perceptual process is the development of definiteness. Hilgard (1951) points out that while stability and definiteness have many common traits they are not identical. To illustrate this distinction he refers to the tendency of the individual to structure visual percepts into figure and ground. This tendency indicates the trend towards 'definiteness' and 'thing quality' (Hilgard, 1951). According to this approach, the individual strives to construct concrete things out of what is perceived, because the concrete is definite in contrast to the conceptual. The perceptual aim of definiteness has adaptive value because it assists the organism to identify objects from minimal environmental signs. The way in which this process may lead to non-veridical perception has already been referred to.

Is the ability to attend and concentrate synonymous with normal cognition? This seems hardly likely in face of the clinical evidence which indicates that in paranoid schizophrenia the capacity to attend may remain intact in spite of cognitive defects affecting thinking and perceiving. However, it is reasonable to assume that defects in conceptual thinking, and loss of stability and definiteness in perception, will inevitably lead to failure in the capacity to attend and concentrate.

In the psychoneurotic patient, visual perception may be influenced in a number of ways and this will lead to a difficulty in attending purposively. Abraham (1913) described the symptoms which may appear in the visual field during the course of a psychoneurotic reaction. In all these instances unconscious phantasies and anxieties interfered with the perceptual process, thus disrupting the patient's capacity to attend to the environment. Complaints of defective concentration which occur commonly enough in the neuroses, independently of visual upsets, are not due to abnormalities of conceptual thinking as such or to a pathology of visual perception. They can generally be traced to the influence of repressed contents upon intact cognitive functions.

Clinical observation suggests that there are, as is so often the case, two forms of disturbance of attention and concentration in mental illness, with a large number of intermediate varieties. In the first type, which is most usually encountered in psychoneurosis and non-psychotic illnesses, the disturbance of attention is the result of the impact of repressed conflicts. In the second type, the attention defect is the end-result of an impairment of cognitive functioning, details of which have already been described earlier in this chapter. This formulation does not exclude the possibility of defects of attending and concentrating in certain psychotic reactions resulting from the influence of repressed conflicts. It is very likely that in those states diagnosed as paranoid psychoses the attention defect is caused both by cognitive deficiencies, as described above, and by repressed conflicts. An explanation such as this takes into account the dynamic and the non-dynamic (organic-functional) factors, both of which must be implicated in mental illnesses of a psychotic nature.

CHAPTER 5

Object Relations and Cognitive Dysfunction

In the last chapter clinical examples were presented demonstrating the disturbances of attention and concentration which may appear in the schizophrenias and paranoid psychoses. In this chapter an attempt will be made to illustrate the connection which exists between cognitive dysfunction and the capacity to relate to others in a meaningful way. The cognitive functions to be examined include the ability to attend purposively, thinking as revealed by the spoken and written word, and perceptual processes. The disorders of perception may appear in the spheres of the self, of the sense of identity, of the body, of sensory modalities and sensation.

Adaptation to the environment and relationship capacity are facets of a unitary process which is 'energized' by neutralized drive (object) cathexes. Adaptation requires that affective reactions be limited in their expression because of their distracting potential and their ability to interfere with the operation of cognitive functions. Affects will follow the vicissitudes of the drive cathexes as the former are regarded as drive derivatives.

The capacity for organized relationships varies considerably in individual psychotic patients. The range extends from those who seem to have lost this capacity completely to others in whom the capacity is well retained. All gradations exist between those two extremes. In this discussion, object-relationship capacity refers to an individual's ability to exhibit organized reaction patterns which are directed towards another person. It is not represented by the diffuse reactivity which can be noted in all psychotic patients, irrespective of the degree of disorganization or withdrawal. Sometimes this non-specific diffuse reactivity is erroneously accorded equal significance with the behaviour designated here as object-relationship capacity (see Chapter 3).

The presence of the object-relationship capacity indicates that the potential to develop genuine transferences is still present. The question to be answered is how varying degrees of loss of the object-relationship capacity correlate with cognitive dysfunction. It is relevant at this point to refer once again to the distinction between the capacity to relate and affective responses. This is necessary because this inquiry is not concerned with the association which may exist between affectivity and cognition. It is solely concerned with investigating how far and in what manner specific cognitive dysfunctions relate to disturbances in object relationships.

A brief account has already been given of the psycho-analytic hypothesis (Chapter 2) that in schizophrenic states there is an alteration in the nature of drive cathexes in the direction of de-neutralization. This theory explains the emergence of uncontrolled libidinal and aggressive tendencies, which are so frequently encountered in schizophrenic patients. Affective reactions of different kinds accompany these manifestations. This hypothesis also states that there is a detachment of the cathexes from the world of objects and their intra-psychic representations. This withdrawal, as has been mentioned above, varies in extent from patient to patient, and cognitive dysfunctions of various kinds occur simultaneously. Two questions arise here: first, what kind of clinical data provide the basis for this psycho-analytic hypothesis, and, second, how do these data reveal connections between the capacity for object relations as described above and cognitive dysfunctions? A start can be made by describing a case in which a severe incapacity for object relations was paralleled by an extensive dysfunction of cognition.

LOSS OF THE OBJECT WORLD AND EXTENSIVE COGNITIVE DYSFUNCTION

CASE 7. The patient was a single woman of thirty-six who had been hospitalized for a period of fourteen years. She had one sister who was mentally healthy. The illness began suddenly with a stream of complaints against her mother. The patient was cruel and aggressive, complaining unceasingly about the mother's behaviour. She was auditorily hallucinated, saying that a man's voice spoke to her and at times there were four voices at once. She felt herself to be under a control. She had to stand in one place or carry out particular instructions. She believed she had unusual strength and power. When first admitted to hospital she told her story well and seemed to make a good

G

contact with the medical and nursing staff. Her illness did not respond to physical treatment and as the months passed she became increasingly withdrawn and inaccessible. Her mental condition remained static over the fourteen-year period without any remission of symptoms. The clinical data detailed below were obtained during two successive interviews, which were part of a sequence of daily sessions held over a period of several months.

Extract from Session A: Interviewer: 'What are you thinking about?' *Patient:* 'She never did like chairs say . . . (she jumped up) . . . I must get out of this office say . . . (she marched up and down the room) . . . I am going to strike you down say . . . I don't know say . . . I would be terribly angry with you say . . . Keep your tongue between your teeth and be terribly angry with you say . . . Do the dirty and I would beat you down say . . . Shout yes for that say . . . My children are like that . . . Yes immediately . . . Sit down Gordon . . . Nan Gordon my favourite sister say . . . He's wasting his time . . . He's wasting his moments. Come off the seat you know he will kill you dead for that . . . Stone dead to the ground to the floor everything . . . Get engaged to me . . . I am sorry to bring you here . . . ' There was some phrase rapidly repeated which was impossible to follow, and she ended up saying: 'Get out of here.' All this was said while walking up and down. Her face was white with rage. *Interviewer:* 'Why are you so angry?' *Patient:* Because I don't like her . . . I hate her . . . She's annoying me . . . She's there beside you . . . I hate her for that . . . You may not do that say . . . If she does that I'll kill her dead into the floor into the ground, everything say . . . '

From this moment she started to march up and down the room and spoke angrily at top speed. *Patient:* 'You can't afford to do that . . . Who the hell is trying to do that . . . You mustn't try to kill anyone . . . Who the hell is she trying to do it to . . . The microphone in this room . . . You mustn't dare to do these things . . . You mustn't dare to kill anyone dead . . . I am going to kill you dead . . . I am going to kill you stone bloody dead today . . . I have no mercy with you, I never had . . . Waste my time . . . (the next phrases were incomprehensible) . . . never do that again . . . Girl never appear here again . . . I can't stand for it. I am not going to sit for it . . . I'm not, I'm not, I'm not . . . She can stick it up her arse . . . ' Among the outpouring the following was recognizable: 'I'll get into a terrible row . . . If she thinks she's going to get away with it . . . I'll get into a terrible row . . . I'll kill you dead

... Fall to the ground ... Gordon ... I never did like her ... Nan Gordon ... and it's all your fault if I don't like my sister ... The secretary of this office ... (she got up from the chair at this moment). Your father beat you up in this room for that say ... Come down say ... I'll kill you dead say ... Sit in the chair and I'm just going to kill you dead for seeing he said. You may not see me say. She's shite that girl say ... Margaret Smith say [the patient's name] ... That gentleman would fleet you.' *Interviewer:* 'What do you mean?' *Patient:* 'Sailor say. Sailor's your wife say ... I don't like you ... No ... I don't like that girl at all say ... She's not a nice girl say ... She's not a nice girl say. (She repeated this several times.) ... I am going to bash you to pulp say ... That girl doesn't like you say ... Get them off the chairs father please ... Can she go out father please? ... She's a bad girl say ... Nan Gordon say ... She would hit you say ... livid say ... (she continued walking up and down) ... (She talked about someone called Blanche in a way impossible to follow) ... I don't like this office say ... (she went to go out). I once hit you for playing at offices ... Your mother say ... Get out of this say ... The child say ... She's always been running away say ... She's a naughty miss say ... Smith was a pain in the bloody arse say. Your mother say ... Shall we go today say? ... Away home say.' She was silent for quite a time and remained sitting on the chair. At this point she slapped herself on the head. *Patient:* 'I hit you for that say ... I hit you just now say ... You were needing hit say ... I had to hit her. She's a bad girl say. She's no use to me. I hit her ... on the ear say ... I had to slap her say. She's a bad girl say.'

Extract from Session B: Before she came into the room she jumped about with rage at the nurse. *Patient:* 'She wants to kill her dead ... She's going to kill me dead say ... Margaret Wilson say ... She is going to kill me dead. My child is one say ... I wouldn't leave it say ... She must go out (went to the door). ... Can she go out now say? ... she's frightened of the chair. She's afraid say ... I'll kill that child dead say ... I must kill her dead say ... Her hair's untidy say ... This child's untidy hair say (she covered the sides of her head with her hands). 'I'm not of their blood say. Too hot in the blood say ... Too hot in the colour say ... Your hair is untidy say ... She's not keeping well today ... The little girl with the fair hair say ... Margaret Smith is your name say ... I am pure white say ... I'll kill her dead say ... It's my father I am looking at say.' (She got up and went to the door.) 'I think we could go down ... father ... I'll need to fix my kilt father ... Can she sew my kilt please?' (She tried to leave the room but agreed to come back.) 'I'll hit you for that say . . . You have to hit this little girl . . . This is a little girl and you have to hit her say . . . I have to hit the little girl say. You must hit her. I can't have that father . . . I fairly go for it say . . . My mother say . . . My mother say . . . I have none say . . . My father say . . . I have none say . . . I am going to beat you up say . . . I'll beat you down proper say . . . I'll beat you to pulp say . . . I need to go now. She's got a sore head.'

The material described above can be examined from the standpoint of the status of the patient's object-relations, the condition of her speech, the extent of perceptual dysfunction, and lastly the ability to attend purposively. In the interviews prior to those in which the above-mentioned data were recorded, the patient was either silent, sitting with her head bowed, or talking rapidly in an angry tone. There was a tendency to incorporate objects in the immediate environment into the content of her utterances. There was no reference to the interviewer. She sometimes obeyed simple commands but was incapable of conducting a rational conversation. She seemed to be indifferent to the interviewer's presence.

The first part of the recorded material was typical of her previous utterances. She was unable to sustain the concept of 'I' and she would change to describing herself in the third person. She was for ever threatening and warning herself. The incident of striking herself reported in Session A showed unequivocally that the 'you' was herself. This reversal and 'turning in on the self' of a drive was a frequent occurrence. 'You' and 'she' on occasions represented the mother, sister, or nurse and finally the material suggested that 'I' also had the significance of the patient's mother. At times it was if the patient was dramatizing an angry scene between mother and child or between mother, sister, and self as adults.

The data revealed an extreme disorder in the form of verbal expression. Although a general theme of hatred directed against the self could be recognized, there was a lack of coherence due to faulty grammatical construction. She was unable to attend to questions asked or statements made by the interviewer. She was at the mercy of her preoccupations or of some external stimulus which was then assimilated into her communications. Words were used incorrectly, as in the phrase 'That gentleman would fleet you'.

The form in which she presented her subjective experiences indicated that she had lost her sense of identity except for brief moments when she gave the impression that 'I' actually referred to herself. Most often she was to be found referring to herself as 'she' or 'that child' or 'S' (her surname). On brief occasions which are not described she referred to herself by the name of another person or as 'Queen Alexandra' or 'the Duke of Edinburgh'. The confusion between 'I', 'she', and 'you' indicated that she had lost the capacity to discriminate herself as an entity from others in the present (nurse, doctor) or from others in the past (mother, sister).

The outbursts of rage that characterized Session A and appeared immediately before Session B were probably stimulated by the interview and the interviewer. The data suggested that she was unwilling to stay in the consulting-room, and many phrases referred to her dislike of having to come or to sit down and talk to the interviewer. It is likely that the introduction of a tape-recorder played a part in the hostile reaction. Although intensely angry, at no time did she direct her rage against the interviewer. When furious about being kept in the room her reaction was, 'You'll have to hit this little girl', thus illustrating her tendency to turn anger in on her self. Apart from a few references to the interviewer or to his secretary, the stage on which the object-relationship drama was acted was that of childhood.

The material reported can be interpreted as a result of transference — that is, as the outcome of a relationship which had arisen between the patient and the interviewer. By displacement the interviewer is equated with mother and the secretary with sister. The rage could be regarded as a result of the jealousy which characterized the triangular relationship of childhood and adolescence (mother, sister, self). While this interpretation takes justifiable account of the patient's capacity to react to the stimulus of the interviewer, it elevates the organizational level on which her mental functioning operates. She was incapable of directing specific and organized reaction patterns to an object outside herself. Everything happened within the confines of the self, which no longer had a boundary.

Objects could not be projected discretely and in sequence onto the person of the interviewer, as would occur in the psycho-analytic therapy of a neurotic patient. She was her childhood self, her mother, and her sister and at the same time her present self, the interviewer, and the secretary. There was no way in which this patient could be made aware of this condensation of past and present. This failure can only be attributed to a complete loss of self-awareness and to an inability to

abstract herself from the immediate situation. She could not discriminate the interviewer as an entity other than one connected with her
childhood as exemplified by the statement, 'Can she go out father
please'.

This patient was capable of reacting to other individuals but her
reaction was diffuse, non-specific, unorganized, uncontrolled, and
without comprehensible latent meaning. Contact with other individuals
intensified the mechanism of turning in on the self. Such a patient is
incapable of developing object relations (transferences) because of the
condensation of self and objects. She cannot attend because attention
demands the presence of object cathexes. At times the content of her
utterances consisted of whatever was within her immediate visual range.
Attention was passive and non-directed, obeying unknown psychic
conditions as, for example, when looking out of the window, she said,
'There is a box. Can I go to get some eggs?' This statement was stimulated by seeing a cardboard box with 'farm eggs' printed on it.

The failure to initiate and sustain object relations ran parallel to
the inability to attend purposively. When this patient was shown a
triangle of matchsticks she could only identify it as three matchsticks and she was unable to reproduce the shape. In this case loss of
the capacity for object relations ran parallel with the severe cognitive
dysfunction affecting attention, speech, thinking, and perceptual discrimination.

THE DELUSION AS A MODE OF OBJECT RELATIONSHIP

CASE 8. The second patient to be described was a woman of forty-five
who had been ill with a schizophrenic illness for a period of nineteen
years. She was married at the time of admission to hospital but was
divorced some years later. At the outset of the illness, which was quite
sudden, she was overactive both physically and mentally. She spoke in a
confused manner and was difficult to follow. The content consisted of
references to sexual misconduct which may have been the cause of
certain self-reproaches. She misidentified the doctor who admitted
her to hospital, confusing her with the wife of the man with whom
she had had an affair. She was hallucinated and expressed a number of
delusional ideas concerning her bodily integrity. She told the admitting
doctor that she (the doctor) had her eyes. This self-object discriminatory
failure was also noted in her delusional belief that she was forced
to have her 'mother's spit'. She would void saliva at this account.

Although initially aggressive and difficult she settled down to life in hospital.

As the data below show, this patient's verbal communications were disordered in their form and characterized by an inability to pursue a theme to its termination. Grammatical defects and neologisms were frequent. At the time of examination the patient presented a rigidly constructed, although simple, delusional complex which consisted of the idea that the headmaster of the school she attended in childhood visited her regularly in hospital and instructed her how to behave in every sphere of living. She no longer responded to her married name and had assumed a new one. There was no impairment in the sense of self. She denied, however, that she had ever been married. She had numerous hypochondriacal delusions and believed that the nurses were men in disguise.

This patient, in spite of these numerous symptoms, was able to undertake useful work in the hospital and was remunerated for it. In certain circumstances, therefore, her capacity to attend and concentrate was not impaired. During the sessions, one of which is described in detail below, she related well to the interviewer and seemed genuinely pleased to see him — having had some contact with him several years previously.

Patient: 'I like working in the garden ... Mr Boyle and Mr Blaney [nurses] take me down. I work in a distillery and in an hotel. I get enough to eat but I would like it better to go home. I sleep without a suck ... a doctor's suck ... ' *Interviewer:* 'What's that?' *Patient:* 'A little bottle; it's got F.L.D.R. on it ... Paraldehyde ... Mr Milne [hallucinatory object — the schoolmaster] wasn't feeling well so I gave him my suck to see if the lift would make Mr Milne sleep ... I'm waiting on the other suck coming in so that I can get to sleep. Yes I gave him mine ... for I was sleeping ... I gave him the lift so that the lift wouldn't go wrong ... The doctor, yet ... was bringing it up.' *Interviewer:* 'The lift?' *Patient:* 'Yes. I didn't want the doctor to be ill or ... stung by the wasps. I don't want the doctor to be ill, saying that he had been stung by the wasps ... ' *Interviewer:* 'Who was stung by the wasps?' *Patient:* 'All the area ... I was stung ... I got saved ... I got cured ... It was the doctor cured — Dr F— [the interviewer] cured it ... Have you passed the bee cure Dr F— ... Have you passed?' *Interviewer:* 'Passed what?' *Patient:* 'To get the cure from the wasps ... Yes ... If not I'll let Mr Milne know to let you get cured ... I mentioned it so that you could get into your proper material ... '

Interviewer: 'Do you see a lot of Mr Milne?' *Patient:* 'Yes thank you.'
Interviewer: 'Does he come into your ward?' *Patient:* 'Yes, He has been
in . . . I am not taken to the wrong area . . . It's the wrong area I am in
. . . I don't like Glasgow. I like South Queensferry . . . He was ever
so nice and the doctor is to be in his class too . . . Dr F— to be in Mr
Milne's class too.

'I wasn't feeling very well doing work in the distillery . . . I think
I am better out of it . . . Better in the garden . . . with Dr F— yes . . .
doctor . . . Mr Milne . . . and Dr F— . . . and Dr F— too if that's if
Dr F— like. I don't speak to them [other people]. They are not in
my with . . . I don't speak to them if they are not my with . . . Mr
Milne wouldn't allow me to speak to them . . . *Interviewer:* 'Why not?'
Patient: 'Because they are not a teacher. Yes . . . passed with the mister
and his with. With Mr . . . Dr F— . . . passed with Mr Milne . . . not
with the wrong teacher.' *Interviewer:* 'What does he say to you?'
Patient: 'Just asked if he was being polite . . . being polite and not staying
away too long.' *Interviewer:* 'When do you hear Mr Milne's voice?'
Patient: 'I hear it every day when I go over to the dit . . . D-I-T.'
Interviewer: 'What is the dit?' *Patient:* 'I go over to stand and see if
Mr Milne's all right, I don't mean to stand in the doctors . . . and then
lie down to go into the doctors, Mr Milne's teaching. I mean not to
stand in the doctors' way. I mean to stand . . . the doctor beside Mr
Milne.' *Interviewer:* 'Where is the dit?' *Patient:* 'Over in the day room.
I have got the lift in. He just asks me if he's not staying away too long.
I say it's all right . . . as long as I get passed to my area . . . and take my
with with me. I had three children, doctor, since I came here and one
of the misses in the day room took them away instead of leaving them
for the sisters to take away . . . Mr Milne.'

This excerpt illustrates how this patient was able, however imperfectly,
to respond to inquiries made by the interviewer. The perceptual
disturbances interfered with her capacity to discriminate environmental
events from her delusional preoccupations and this added to the incoherence of her communications. The speech disorder was not limited
to grammatical errors but words were also used concretely and had the
significance of real objects (for example 'with'). Striking clinical features were the tendency to misidentify and the failure to discriminate
the self from objects. This patient confused the interviewer with the
delusional object (the schoolmaster) and also with herself. The statement about the cure from the bee sting illustrated this condensation

clearly. Periodically she failed to distinguish the interviewer from the ward sister and in general she had difficulty in discriminating men from women. This manifestation is not uncommon in schizophrenic states, probably being due to the projected conflict over sexual identity. In contrast to Case 7, this patient retained the sense of self and always referred to herself in the first person.

This patient differed from Case 7 in so far as she could attend to simple tasks and could participate in a conversation although, as already mentioned, her utterances were often difficult to follow. The ability to attend was associated with a limited capacity for relationships, which was reflected in the content of the delusional system. Her condensation of the interviewer and the delusional object was another instance of her tendency to fuse the delusional object with individuals who were important in her immediate environment. The ward sister and the head gardener were two such persons.

This case demonstrates that it is wrong to envisage delusional complexes as necessarily rigid, unchanging, or without purpose. Though delusions arise as a result of purely endopsychic events, once they have appeared they can be of vital importance in the patient's life. In this patient's case the delusional complex was malleable and was utilized for purposes of adaptation to hospital life. Changing circumstances led to an alteration in the manner in which the content presented itself. This case is not an exception among long-stay schizophrenic patients. Further examples of the manner in which delusional content can alter when confronted with new environmental stimuli are described in Chapter 7.

SPEECH DISTURBANCE AS A MEASURE OF OBJECT-RELATIONS CAPACITY

Cases 7 and 8 stimulate interest in the nature of the speech disturbance in the schizophrenias and how much significance is to be attributed to this disorder as an index of overall mental dysfunction. It is always necessary to remember that it is only through the observation of the defects in verbalization that the observer can gain an insight into the state of the thought processes. Psycho-analytic studies have generally supported Bleuler's (1911) contention that the disorder of verbalization in the schizophrenias is a secondary phenomenon. This deficiency arises from a basic fault in the processes which lead to conceptual thinking and thus to meaningful verbal communication.

The speech defects of Cases 7 and 8 can be compared, first, by examining the form of the verbal utterances and, second, by inspecting the nature of the content. In both instances alterations in the form of speech were to be noted. The construction of phrases and sentences was defective and grammatical rules were not observed. It was, however, in the sphere of content that the most striking differences between the two patients occurred. In Case 7 the content rarely varied and was monotonously repeated. The perseverative tendency in speech was also to be observed in writing and in the course of attempting to carry out simple tasks. The material suggests that in these two patients a speech defect existed alongside the disorder of thinking. The former found expression in faulty syntax and perseveration, the latter in condensations, concretization, and magic thinking.

It may be surmised that Case 7 was incapable of creating the psychic representation of an object distinct from herself. She was both part of the objects of her childhood and part of their adult counterparts. In the second case, object cathexes were invested in the delusional object and as a consequence of the perceptual defects real persons became fused with the delusional object. Although this patient failed at times to discriminate herself clearly as an entity from other entities, she still had a residual capacity for relating, even though this only found delusional expression. This woman's delusions and hallucinations were a substitute for real objects — restitutional products — to employ the classical psycho-analytic terminology.

Comparison of the two patients suggests the the difference in the speech disturbance lay principally in the content rather than in the abnormality of form. Does this mean that the content of a schizophrenic patient's utterances can be regarded as a measure of the object-relationship capacities, even though these capacities may lead only to delusion formation rather than to real relationships with others? Little emphasis can be placed on disturbance of the form of speech alone, since hospitalization effects and the lack of conversational opportunities may play a large part in faulty grammatical construction in chronic patients. Opportunities for conversation sometimes lead to a striking improvement in the form of the patient's speech. Again, disorders of speech form are extremely common in acute psychotic breakdowns which have a good prognosis. Defective speech form will be of more sinister significance when it appears together with an extreme degree of withdrawal from the environment and with the absence of organized delusional ideas.

For the present the appearance of delusional objects has been taken as indicating the presence of some kind of capacity for relationships. The cathexes which operate in such instances must be regarded as distinct from the neutralized object cathexes which provide the foundation for object relationships in the mentally healthy. They are, at best, object cathexes of narcissistic type.

These deluded patients are not entirely divorced from their environment and they can make some kind of adaptation to others. Does this mean, as the classical psycho-analytical theory would maintain, that residual neutralized object cathexes remain intact, operating alongside those (? narcissistic) cathexes which appear to 'energize' the delusional object? Clinical observation supports this hypothesis, because of the impression that these patients are operating on two different levels. Often they are rational in their utterances and in their contact with others, whereas at other times they are dominated by delusional preoccupations.

Both Bleuler and Freud regarded the disorder of thinking in the schizophrenias as a secondary reaction. If so, then fluctuations in thought content will depend upon the state of the primary disturbance. An index of the primary disturbances could therefore be the capacity to relate. On this account it is important to inquire into how far defects in this capacity are associated with faults in thinking as reflected in speech. What kind of speech form and content is to be found in schizophrenic patients with well-organized and coherent delusional systems that allow them to make a kind of relationship with objects?

FORM AND CONTENT OF SPEECH ASSOCIATED WITH ORGANIZED DELUSIONS

CASE 9. The patient was an unmarried man of fifty-three who had been ill with paranoid schizophrenia for approximately twenty years. His first period of hospitalization was in 1947. It lasted for about one year. At that time he had grandiose and persecutory delusions. He believed he was composed of several persons — a kind of composite individual. He was under the impression that his body has been made lighter and had been changed in shape. His visual perceptual function was disordered with respect to size constancy. After discharge from hospital he remained at home for about eight years, still entertaining his delusional ideas. His condition deteriorated, however, and he had to be hospitalized again in 1956 and has remained so since that time. He continued to present a grandiosity and omnipotence which the material detailed below will illustrate. There was never any loss in the sense of identity nor was the construction of his speech seriously distorted. In the following excerpt the patient tells the interviewer how a criminal band operates through the patients and staff of the hospital.

Excerpt from Interview: Interviewer: 'How are you keeping?' *Patient:* 'Very good . . . I am fifty-three now . . . I am very fit . . . I can run about and play football . . . I play with the children sometimes . . . I do a lot of walking about the grounds . . . It is very healthy walking about the grounds . . . especially amongst the fields and trees and flowers . . . and how are you doing yourself? . . . You look very well . . . you seem to be growing stronger . . . getting stronger looking . . . your top shoulders are stronger looking . . . You're growing quite a big strong man.'

He was asked why he carried a little sack around with him and he said it was because there were so many thieves in the hospital. *Patient:* ' . . . Every night thieves get the keys of the cupboards and rummage through all the lockers . . . '*Interviewer:* 'Are all the patients the victims of these thieves?' *Patient:* 'No . . . they are not so much victims, only you could regard them as victims . . . they are the very highest for the use of . . . they are the highest tools these thieves have to use . . . the tools they use are human beings . . . people and they "per" them . . . ' *Interviewer:* What does that mean?' *Patient:* 'The people seem to do . . . the lunatics seem to do . . . They go out and thieve . . . They move them about like puppets . . . like puppets on a string they do it per them . . . You never meet these thieves you meet their tools . . . their tools are all men and women . . . The ones in here are the very highest . . . There is no crime that is ever done that is not done "per" them . . . But it's done subtly . . you can try and watch . . . that great train robbery was done "per" your patients here . . . and nobody else . . . ' *Interviewer:* 'How did they get down there?' *Patient:* 'They didn't go down, it goes out from them to other people outside . . . to other people, by affinity and similarity and sympathy . . . They carried it on from one to another one . . . They are puppeting all the time . . . Not one of them was a thief, not a criminal . . . Scotland Yard learned this — you must have had sympathy for them. They are only the seeming thieves . . . Starts off from here . . . The lunatics do nothing they merely are "for the use of" . . . It all starts with the male nurses . . . '

Interviewer: 'What do they do?' *Patient:* 'Nothing ... The male nurses, then the patients ... people outside ... visitors ... male nurses, patients, visitors ... official visitors ... Then people outside who have never met ...' *Interviewer:* 'How does the message get from one to another?' *Patient:* 'By slips – by slipism automation ... some remote time – an umpteen multiplied by an umpteen years ago ... Very brainy and clever ... They are very brainy criminals ... nothing like these people ... Slipism ... They invite you to their house ... then they dope you and they cut up your body and they make slips of you and they "cannibalize" and suck the rest and guts it ... guts it and take it and pack it around their own flesh and their own body ... They were very delicate criminals ... Very greatest of doctors and surgeons ... That's been carried on like that and these people that puppet ... The puppets have to show their slipism, the hair-blood and body-slip of you – the male nurses, the lunatics are their own persons, but they put it on by invisible strings – motivated automation by water, electricity, gas, and as many other such powers as can be added and they have the affinity and the sympathy ... Slipism is the whole key – without slipism they can't do it ... they suck the blood ... take the whole flesh and blood and body over and make it up to look like Dr F– [interviewer] and put it on strings and work it ... They put the slips from the nurse into the patient – it's two ways ... From the nurse to the patient, from the patient to the nurse and they drape it around their back – you can see an awful lot of men's jackets like this ... They stick up an awful lot at the back (interviewer's jacket was so affected) ... Sticking up in an unusual, para-normal way ... They put the slips from the nurses into the patient ... The patient into the male nurse and they also drape him around the back of the head like a sort of frame ... They keep working continuously – one to the other ... The slip is a mere reflection of a man ...'

'It's going done [criminal influence] ... At a rapid rate ... You will find that people will grow much better ... Also with better complexions and look better and be much slimmer ... They will lose these great bellies and backsides ... That's all criminal stuff ... All puppetry.' *Interviewer:* 'Do you say that if the slips were done away with people would be much healthier?' *Patient:* 'Yes, because the slips die back into your body ... You can call it "die" or you can call it "live" ... The slip merges into your body ... Much healthier because they have got all that back into their own body ... The slips are made of hair-blood and body stuff ... You get them all back into your body ...

You [interviewer] would grow hair on your head again . . . You won't need glasses . . . Myopia is caused by too much strain being put this way and that way and blurred vision.' *Interviewer:* 'Do things change their shape?' *Patient:* 'No you don't see the correct shape . . . . Everybody is distorted — everybody looks utterly unlike themselves.' *Interviewer:* 'Different identity?' *Patient:* 'Yes . . . it gives them a different appearance and a different identity . . . '

Interviewer: 'Do they affect you?' *Patient:* 'I am immune to it . . . I never got host hospitality . . . They never gave me host hospitality because I have got a distrusting nature . . . You can be as kind and gentle and cheerful and well-spoken . . . I was always sceptical . . . I agree with Shakespeare — all men are liars and all men are rotters. I am not.

This excerpt illustrates the very essence of magic thinking as described by Frazer (1890) in the *Golden Bough*. Causal relationships are assumed on the basis of similarity and temporal contiguity as in the statement ' . . . to other people by affinity and similarity and sympathy'. The form of this patient's verbal utterances was intact, but it was the content which provided insight into the quality of the patient's relationships. This man was prepared to come to interviews and he expressed himself freely as the material illustrates. In this respect he differed entirely from withdrawn, negativistic patients.

It was through the delusional ideas that this patient's inner feelings about others emerged although in a disguised form. The delusion was a channel for communicating with other individuals in the same manner as Case 8. Much of what he expressed through the delusions indicated his supreme contempt for doctors and nurses. In the following quotation he indirectly expressed his superiority in perceptiveness and exposed the limitations of the interviewer. This statement showed that it was the psychiatrist who was controlled and under influence and not himself.

Patient: 'You're speaking just now . . . You're using your mouth, you weren't yesterday morning . . . Somebody was speaking through you yesterday morning . . . Someone was interfering with your speech . . . There is no interference just now.' *Interviewer:* 'How do you detect that?' *Patient:* 'It's simple you watch them . . . Their mouths don't move . . . The speech comes from here or there as they show you in the cartoons in the newspaper . . . It comes from their feet . . . The deep voice as if it came from the soles of their feet . . . It can come from their fingers . . . '

His infinite superiority to the interviewer is made manifest in the following excerpt. (He began mouthing words without any sound emerging. He was asked what he was doing.) *Patient:* 'Speaking to a man behind you...' *Interviewer:* 'Do you see him?' *Patient:* 'Yes ... He's another man of you... He's very like you... I was telling him that these people of the Den [the hospital] the staff and the lunatics — the highest for the use of...' *Interviewer:* 'How did the man get there?' *Patient:* 'He's there all the time... He's there all the time... He's a familiar of you... Have you never heard of a man having familiars?... Every man has familiars...' *Interviewer:* 'A double?' *Patient:* 'You could argue he's your double... He's just like you in appearance... He's a double of you in appearance in disguise... He's another man of you... The more familiars a man has the more successful he will be...' *Interviewer:* 'What do these familiars do?' *Patient:* 'All sorts of things to help you... They strive all the time to keep you from slipism automation... That's why you are as free as you are... The abler a man's familiars, the freer you will be... Your name indicates that you have been a blackman... You have been a blackman and a slave... First of all you won your freedom from slavery — maybe in the U.S.A. — then you freed slaves. Then you got rid of this blackness and for all practical purposes, though not completely and fully, you got rid of slipism and automation and became a man so you got the name F—... Most men given themselves their own name... The criminals assist you to give yourself a name... The name F— to show to all of them to leave you alone... You have a job for life — a doctor of the dennery [the hospital]... In another hundred years your senses will be as alert as mine and you will not use the name F—... You'll be far more free and you will not use the name then... You'll use some other name... You'll be undoubtedly free then.'

These data can be interpreted as resulting from the activity of the mechanism described as denial in phantasy (A. Freud, 1936), which is so common in childhood. In this particular instance the patient repressed disturbing bodily experiences which characterized the early phases of the illness. He now perceived them as affecting the interviewer. He reversed the distressing inner and outer reality for something more agreeable. This was accomplished by omnipotence and magical thinking. Yet this defence was not completely successful because there remained a dread of the interviewer (the result of a projection of destructive phantasies) as is revealed in the following statement:

Patient: 'You can see your desk top so that the watch isn't there at all
... It's merged into the appearance of the desk ... It's called lunatic's
delusion. They see you looking as the most demoniacal character ...
They are terrified and you are the doctor – their only help. You have
got to give them psychiatric treatment. They so shrink back they're
terrified. You look such a demoniacal character ... You cannot help
them – it stops the therapy being successfully accomplished.'

The clinical phenomena presented support the view already elaborated
that there are patients who employ their delusional ideas as a bridge to
the world of objects. In these patients (Cases 8 and 9) speech may be
intact or disordered in its form. The content of the delusions, although
internally consistent, is based on magical thinking – on omnipotence of
thought. In patients such as Case 9, verbal symbols retain their structure
and the neutralized cathexes necessary for expressing and comprehend-
ing meaning, but the organizational level of thinking has fallen into a
state which is less concerned with external realities than with the inner
psychic reality. Running parallel with this condition of thought is a
precarious hold on the real world maintained through the delusional
complex.

When the verbal capacity is preserved it is sometimes easy to discern
latent themes in the patient's utterances. These latent thoughts are
usually provoked by the stimulus of the interview situation. Anxieties
about reactions to the interviewer lead some psychotic patients to find
a devious expression for their thoughts. It would appear as if they are
unable, in contrast to psychoneurotic patients who may have similar
reactions, to repress their ideational and affective responses adequately.
Thus they have recourse to less stable defences such as regression,
denial, and reversal. When the stress is relieved the defence is superfluous and verbal communication is restored to a normal level. When the
defence is expressed through the medium of speech it seems as if the
patient has a private language (Burnham, 1955) whose meaning is
unknown to outsiders. Its very obscurity protects the patient against
the risk of being slighted or rebuffed and simultaneously denies feelings
of helplessness through the grandiosity of its content.

Those who have studied or treated schizophrenic patients psycho-
therapeutically have often commented on this fact – namely that
formal aspects of speech fluctuate between the normal and the abnormal
condition. They have also suggested, as Cameron does in Chapter 10,
that it is possible to understand the content of the patient's utterances

as reflecting aspects of his feelings about the therapeutic relationship. While these assertions seem justified in many cases, they may not apply to all patients suffering from schizophrenic illnesses. There are a great number of chronic schizophrenic patients who show a most extensive and unchanging disorganization of speech and thinking. When these patients speak, their conversation consists of isolated and disconnected words or phrases. There is little trace of grammatical construction, making the phenomenon almost indistinguishable from jargon or agrammatical dysphasia (Schilder, 1928b). The patient often fails to understand written or spoken words. McGhie points out in Chapter 9 that this difficulty in speech comprehension possibly results from '... a deficiency in perceiving the words in meaningful relationship to each other as part of an organized pattern'. Paraphasic phenomena can also be observed in this group of patients (Curran & Schilder, 1935).

The case described below is typical of this group of patients.

PERSISTENCE OF JARGON SPEECH (AGRAMMATISM) IN PSYCHOSIS

CASE 10. This patient was a single man of twenty-nine who was admitted to hospital at the age of nineteen. He had fallen ill while in the Army. The illness appeared to have been precipitated by a disappointment. At the onset of the illness his capacity to communicate was badly impaired. He was confused and mixed up — beginning to speak and then breaking off in the middle of a sentence. The content of his speech was incoherent. He expressed fleeting persecutory and omnipotent ideas. He remained in hospital for one year, being discharged with little improvement. Two years later he was readmitted as his mental state had deteriorated. He was now inaccessible, although there were occasions when he was mentally and physically overactive. The following excerpt which followed immediately after an electro-shock treatment illustrates the state of his verbal communications.

Interviewer: 'How are you feeling?' *Patient:* '...I slept with thirty thousand million people in my time...I had a brain operation... and a couple of... punched my nose in. About six thousand years ago. For censorship of the authorization... of fair hair... anti-strong men ...Building things... Renewing perhaps...If you philosophize... A piece of a tenement...If you don't know what it's called...A fractice people...to burial junk...isn't it?...How does it cost?...' *Interviewer:* 'What?' *Patient:* 'The paternity fees...Is his fee arranged?

H

... Building ... How are you feeling ... How are you feeling? ...
Brain ... Oh, are you in hospital ... Are they going to operate on
your brain for a spell ... Leave you the cat to carry ... Practicational
retirement ... Yes, you see, that's what happens to most causes ...
Take it off and leave it ...' *Interviewer:* 'Take what off?' *Patient:*
'Your brain off and leave you casually sadistic ... Yes, quite ... How
are you feeling? ... And you take it and you take it off ... Play with it
... People play with your brain at operations ... You have got a perfect ... operations sadistical ... You should know it back down perhaps ... You've got such a perfect brain ... with lying idle.' *Interviewer:* 'Who's got such a perfect brain?' *Patient:* 'Everyone has it
at times but I've got a distorted brain ... Perhaps I was born in the work-
house ... Born ... Five ... If you knock the essential building down
... Well if you look up it's the whole ... Knocks the building down
and lets himself in ... Occasional practical ... How are you feeling?
... Are you the heart specialist? ... Are you the ... My paternal
way ... Habitation ... Operation in me ... Sabbatical systematic
continuation of this thing ... Start operating on the brain ... Take it
off and give them practical tardation ... Yes about fifteen thousand
million years perhaps ... Kill them may be ... Practically sleeping,
Christ knows ... Traditional ... Practical medicine ... Yes there's
theological and independence ... I have lost all doctors' education.'

In this illustration, apart from the reference to reactions to the electro-
shock treatment, there was no means of knowing what the patient
was specifically trying to communicate. His utterances were fragmented,
unstructured, perseverative, and characterized by echo-reactions (echo-
lalia). They remained in this state over a period of many years. This is
a common experience in mental hospital practice. There are patients of
this type whose hospitalization continues for long periods and who are
never heard to speak in a logical or coherent manner. In cases of this
kind the organizational level of thinking cannot be thought of as similar
to a developmental phase of childhood thinking or with the thinking of
primitives, as can the content of other psychotic patients – for example,
Case 9. In these deteriorated states words are used without their having
any reference to things or to concepts which have a validity in the
world of experience. The fragmentation which affects speech and
thinking also occurred in the realm of object relationships.

Phenomena of this kind indicate how words may lose their symbolic
function. In these deteriorated cases words are no longer used as in-

struments for the expression or comprehension of thought. Psycho-analysis explains such pathological phenomena as the result of words having become cathected with instinctual energy and then used for purposes other than communication. The extent to which this disorganization of speech and thinking proceeds varies from patient to patient and as a rule it is accompanied by a complete withdrawal of object cathexes.

Freud (1911) must have had patients of this kind in mind when he suggested that in cases of dementia praecox there is a regression of the libido (instinctual cathexes) to the phase of auto-erotism — that is, to an infantile period before objects existed. This concept of a return to auto-erotism in dementia praecox describes a state where the patient has abandoned the world of objects and the means of entering into a relationship with them. Words, having lost their correct function, are now employed auto-erotically in the service of the instinctual drives. In these deteriorated states efforts to regain contact with objects is limited to hallucination. In such cases auditory and visual hallucinations are transitory in nature, and there is an absence of organized delusional complexes of even the most simple kind.

In these disintegrated states, object cathexes have been completely disorganized and have regained their instinctual quality. The cathexes are no longer directed to objects and therefore there is no capacity for transference. This view is not accepted by many psycho-analysts (Rosenfeld, 1952; Searles, 1963a), and their technique of treatment is based upon consistent attention to a latent transference which they assume is present (see Chapters 3 and 10).

In deluded patients (Cases 8 and 9) the delusions themselves express the activity of cathexes directed towards objects. These cathexes are instinctual in nature and show characteristics of the organization which is described as the phase of primary narcissism. The idea of self exists, but objects are not clearly differentiated from this embryonic self. At this phase mental functioning is governed by the primary process. This hypothesis is based upon those deluded patients who relate to the world through their delusional objects which are narcissistic in nature. The activity of the primary process can be inferred from the discriminatory defects which characterize thinking and perceiving.

THEORETICAL INFERENCES

The clinical evidence from both acute and chronic cases favours the hypothesis that there is a close connection between a patient's capacity for relationships and the state of the thought processes as revealed through speech form and content. Delusional complexes, when they appear, enable a patient to form a kind of object relationship and this is some-times achieved through a condensation of the real object with a phan-tasy object belonging to the delusion itself – for example, Case 8. Thus the patient may come to relate to the physician or nurse in either a positive or a negative way. These relationships are based on instinctual (narcissistic) cathexes governed by the primary-process mechanisms of condensation and displacement. They are qualitatively distinct from the neutralized cathexes which operate in the non-psychotic individual. The form of speech and thinking cannot alone be taken as an index of a cathectic withdrawal from objects.

Similar considerations apply to the perceptual disorders which are frequently encountered in different psychotic syndromes. A severe discriminatory incapacity in the self-object sphere does not imply an inability to relate. Many acute cases which follow a favourable course show defects in self-object discrimination alongside intense object-seeking behaviour (Freeman, 1962a). Greater significance is to be attri-buted to perception of the self and sense of identity as prognostic indices. If the sense of identity is lost, there is also loss of the object world. Partial defects in the sense of identity are to be found concomitantly with the retention of some capacity for object relations. This was so in Case 8. Disturbance in size and distance constancies and synaesthestic phenomena are of less significance as indices of derangement of object relations, occurring as they do in so many different forms of schizo-phrenic and non-schizophrenic illness.

The data provided by deteriorated states (Cases 7 and 10) suggest that there is a category of schizophrenic patients in which speech, thinking, and perceptual dysfunction are primary in nature. The group of patients is characterized by an abandonment of the object world and its psychic representations – by a complete loss of the sense of self and identity and by a disorganization of speech and thinking. This hypothesis is supported by the observation that, once this series of clinical mani-festations is firmly established, it never shows a movement towards normality – a movement which is so frequently encountered, even if only transiently, in other psychotic patients showing less severe forms of cognitive dysfunction. The experimental findings reported by McGhie in Chapter 9 also point to a primary cognitive defect in certain cases of schizophrenia.

From a review of the clinical data that have been described in this chapter, it becomes apparent that the ability to attend purposively, speech, conceptual thinking, and perceptual discrimination will be deranged in varying degrees paralleling the extent of the object-relationship disturbance. Psycho-analytic theory lays stress on the dysfunction of the cathectic processes as a means of explaining the phenomena encountered in psychotic states. Not only it there a failure of conceptual thinking owing to the intrusion of a more primitive form of cathectic 'energy' — the primary process — where condensation and displacement predominate, but in addition, as Rosen (1953) has suggested, the de-cathexis of irrelevant contents necessary for conceptual thought in all its different aspects does not occur. Attention has already been drawn to the fact that neurophysiologists utilize the idea of a failure of inhibition to explain this category of phenomenon.

In cases of paranoid psychosis the failure of concept formation is minimal, and it is only moderately impaired in those patients in whom there is a fairly well-organized delusional complex. It is implicit in the classical psycho-analytic theory of psychosis that the delusion protects against further deterioration of cognitive functions. Defects in concept formation and perceptual upsets are usually limited in paranoid psychoses to the content of the delusion. The clinical evidence favours the hypothesis that an association exists between delusion formation, on the one hand, and the level at which cognitive functions operate, on the other. Better-preserved cognition is associated with more sophisticated delusional content.

This clinically based hypothesis is further strengthened by the observation that in patients manifesting a delusional complex there is some retention of the object-relationship capacity and the ability to attend purposively. This can be understood as resulting from a restraint being imposed upon the further intrusion of the primary process into the whole sphere of mental functioning. This restraint is absent in the hebephrenias, where condensation characterizes thinking, perception, and object relationships. It is in these states that loss of identity, severe incapacity, and abandonment of object relations occur.

The study of deluded patients shows that the delusions have important adaptive functions. They are vehicles for the establishment of communications with the real world. It is surely not by chance that the patients who are without delusional complexes are generally fragmented, isolated, and withdrawn. Cases 7 and 10 are good examples of this. While the nucleus of a delusion remains constant and influences the perception of environmental events the remaining content is not necessarily inalterable. Additions and deletions can take place depending upon external circumstances.

Delusional complexes could be said to differ in terms of the rigidity of their boundary. In some cases the boundary is extremely permeable permitting the assimilation of new impressions or experiences. In other instances it is fixed, resisting the impact of fresh environmental stimulation. An analogy could be made between the behaviour of delusions and that of the semi-permeable membrane. Their functional core consists of the selective transmission of contents both extrinsic and intrinsic. They are equally sensitive to the slightest changes in their own content or in the medium in which they may be placed. Such changes are reacted to in the manner that will be least damaging to the physical or psychological system. Essentially both have a homeostatic function. This analogy is only useful in so far as it draws attention to the dynamic nature of the delusion, even when it appears to be petrified and immutable. It comes to mind at once that delusions with fixed boundaries and contents are more commonly found in patients who are persecuted and very afraid.

The large number of psychotic patients whose mental disturbance remits spontaneously or with the aid of treatment certainly adds support to the classical theory that all the major manifestations of the schizophrenias are secondary phenomena. Every experienced psychiatrist has encountered acute schizophrenic patients in whom thinking disorder, defects in the identity sense, loss of the object world, and various perceptual dysfunctions have characterized the clinical state, and yet therapy or the passage of time has led to the disappearance of all these phenomena.

This suggests that the mental processes of schizophrenic patients always retain the potential for maximal function. This view is only contradicted by the existence of those chronic patients in whom there is never any restoration of function. It was proposed on the basis of these observations and the results obtained by McGhie and Chapman (see Chapter 9) that there may be a group of states (formerly designated dementia praecox) in which there is a central defect manifesting itself in primary symptoms comprising loss of the object world, loss of identity, and loss of the verbal capacity. Apart from time, the only index that might differentiate between the benign and the malignant case is the patient's capacity to relate as revealed in a psychotherapeutic relationship. The slightest ability to react in an organized and specific way to the impact of the therapist may be of greater prognostic significance than defects in visual perception or loss of self-object discrimination.

The view has been advanced in this chapter that psychotic symptomatology, particularly as it appears in the sphere of cognition, must not be assessed in isolation but must be examined alongside a scrutiny of the patient's capacity for object relationships and thus the state of the underlying cathexes. Psycho-analytic experience demonstrates that all psychotic patients are sensitive to stimuli that arise from contact with others. In many cases (for example, Case 7) these reactions are but the disorganized remains of what once was an ability to enter into a human relationship with its implications of mutual influence and concern. What must be determined is whether or not the patient retains, even in the smallest degree, the capacity for relations with an individual outside himself. This capacity may appear only transiently and be impaired by difficulties in self-discrimination. Nevertheless, its very presence is indicative of a potential for transference.

The general non-specific reactivity of psychotic patients cannot be regarded as an expression of object-libidinal cathexes and such phenomena must be differentiated from the ability to relate to objects in the environment. Insufficient distinction has been drawn in the case of psychotic reactions between diffuse reactivity, on the one hand, and organized reaction patterns, on the other. This has led to confusing patients whose cognitive functions will remain permanently disorganized and fragmented with those in whom the same functions can return to normal in a short period of time. It has led to pessimism regarding the possibility of differentiating psychotic states on the basis of symptomatology alone. This is not necessarily so, if the differentiating criterion is the capacity for object relationships as defined earlier in this book and in this chapter.

CHAPTER 6

The Nature and Function of Hallucinations

Hallucinatory phenomena are frequently encountered in functional psychoses. From a diagnostic standpoint considerable significance is given to auditory hallucinations as a criterion of a schizophrenic illness in contrast to visual hallucinations, which occur in various forms of functional and organic psychosis. Nevertheless, visual hallucinations are not uncommon in the hebephrenias alongside auditory hallucinations. They are rare in the paranoid variety of the illness. In the textbooks written by an earlier generation of psychiatrists it was common to encounter the concept of the hysterical hallucination. These perceptual anomalies — in both the auditory and visual spheres — were thought of as being an aspect of a severe neurotic disorder which had to be distinguished from the functional psychoses and the milder neurotic reactions.

Today it is uncommon to hear or read about hysterical hallucinations. It is more usual to regard the appearance of auditory hallucinations as the expression of a schizophrenic reaction. The view adopted here is that the appearance of hallucinatory phenomena results from the derangement of the function which enables the individual to discriminate between thoughts and images, on the one hand, and perceptual experience, on the other hand. It is also believed that the mechanism underlying hallucinatory phenomena is identical whatever the diagnostic category. Other factors operate to produce the clinical phenomena that characterize the condition as one of nuclear schizophrenia (dementia praecox), schizophreniform psychosis, paranoid schizophrenia, paranoid psychosis, or hysterical psychosis — the diagnosis depending upon the clinician's diagnostic orientations.

The hypothesis outlined below follows from the psycho-analytic theory of hallucinations, a reference to which was made in Chapter 2. Freud's (1900) first explanations of hallucination followed from his study of dreams. He pointed out that the essential feature in the dream was the conversion of memory traces into visual percepts (hallucinations). In waking life this transformation is impossible for the mentally healthy, no matter how vivid or compelling the memory trace or imagery. Hallucinatory phenomena may be regarded as similar to the manifest dream — memory traces, images, and verbal ideas can be experienced as percepts.

In order to provide an explanation for the transformation of an image or a memory trace into a percept, Freud (1900) had recourse to his concept of the mental apparatus 'energized' by cathexes of different kinds. It is irrelevant here to engage in controversy over the value of utilizing such concepts, with their connotation of energy transformation (free-bound cathexis) and distribution within the nervous system (Holt, 1962). Of greater importance is the psychological conception of different classes and forms of mental organization which are capable of transposition from one level of complexity to another. The terms used to describe and explain such changes (primary and secondary process; condensation and displacement) are essentially explanatory (psychological) concepts and need not describe the actual mechanics of the underlying physiological processes. All agree with the view that the cause of the hallucinatory and dream phenomena will eventually be found in the physico-chemical activity of the nervous system. At the present the time the psychological approach, with its inevitably vague and inexact concepts, must be employed until such knowledge is obtained.

Hallucinations in clear consciousness are explained by psychoanalytic theory in a similar manner to that described for the dream. The simplest form of hallucination arises from wishful phantasies. The ideational content is activated by drive 'energy' (instinctual cathexes) and, as a consequence of the disease process, phantasies or discrete images come to be experienced as visual or auditory percepts (hallucinations). The concept of topographic regression, as employed here, is the basic mechanism underlying the hallucinatory process, just as in the case of dream formation. Freud's contribution to the understanding of hallucinatory experience was his discovery that these phenomena (hallucinations) arise initially in relation to objects of significance to the individual patient. In the following illustration it is possible to follow the development of hallucination *in statu nascendi*.

HALLUCINATIONS AS THE REACTION TO
AN OBJECT-RELATIONSHIP CONFLICT

CASE 11. The patient was a single woman of twenty-eight who complained of depression of mood, irritability, and fatigue. When she was first seen, there was nothing to suggest the presence of a psychotic reaction. The patient had been ill initially when she was twenty-six years old. She was admitted to a mental hospital because of unpredictable behaviour. At that time there was a fear that she might be suffering from a schizophrenic illness. She had been having difficulties at university and this led to failure in examination. In her second year she fell in love with a lecturer, and disappointment in this respect was accompanied by depression of mood, non-attendance at classes, and difficult relations at home.

When she failed to get her degree she left home and worked in another city. On her return, it was noted that her behaviour had changed. She was alternately elated and dejected, and then tearful, self-critical, and agitated. She remained in her room for long periods and her personal habits deteriorated. After a month or two had passed, she agreed to undertake a teacher-training course, but unfortunately she came in contact with the lecturer with whom she had been infatuated. This led to deterioration in her mental state. She remained in a depressed condition for a number of months and, since the condition did not improve, she was recommended to enter a mental hospital.

On admission to hospital at the age of twenty-six, she showed no sign of formal thought disorder, delusions, or hallucinations. She admitted to acting on impulse and continued with her self-criticism and self-reproach. Within a matter of weeks the depressive symptoms disappeared and she was discharged from hospital. For a year following discharge she undertook a teacher-training course and when it was completed taught for one year, but during this time found herself in low spirits. She lost confidence in herself and had little interest in work. It was on this account that she was again referred for a psychiatric opinion and on this occasion she was offered outpatient psychotherapy. There was no reason at this time to suspect the presence of a psychotic illness. Outpatient treatment continued for four years until she had to be readmitted to a mental hospital at the age of thirty-two.

The psychotherapeutic process can, for the purpose of description, be divided into three phases. The first phase was characterized symptomatologically by depressive manifestations. The self-criticisms were initially confined to performance at work, but later they found an outlet in other spheres — particularly in the treatment situation. During the first phase the patient developed an intense positive transference. She expressed her love and admiration for the therapist. Her idealization showed that this transference was essentially narcissistic in nature. He was merely the vehicle for her latent self-admiration. She believed that the therapist had abilities and attributes quite beyond his real capacity and she consistently refused to examine the basis for her beliefs.

Within a short time she began to express concern for the therapist's health and welfare. She was constantly worrying in case she annoyed or upset him. She would scrutinize his appearance whenever possible. She was concerned lest her case should impose too great a strain and make him ill. Throughout this period she did everything that she thought might please the therapist. This patient had no difficulty whatever in expressing irritation with her mother and her belief that she had been unwanted. Ventilation of death wishes towards her mother and a sister who was five years younger led to some alleviation of the depression. Work at school improved and her adjustment seemed to be better. There was, however, no change in the narcissistic nature of the transference. Considerable attention was directed to the analysis of defences based upon introjection, but without beneficial result. The patient had firmly internalized the therapist and the destructive phantasies that were directed against him. Through the mechanism of isolation the patient was able to keep the therapist good and the mother bad. At the same time projection of superego attitudes onto the therapist led to a fear of being criticized.

Holidays were times of difficulty for the patient. She was usually depressed and worried about what the therapist would be doing. She was able to phantasy about his holiday activities but never at any time expressed dissatisfaction at being left. Towards the end of the first phase of the treatment, which lasted for three years, she brought confirmation of the narcissistic phantasies which her behaviour and utterances had suggested. She said for a long time she had been convinced that the improvement in her condition and in her life circumstances was due to an actual intervention by the therapist. She believed that he had spoken to the headmaster of her school and had made arrangements for her to find good lodgings.

Little progress was made in removing the resistance of idealization. However, material was obtained that threw light on phases of her early childhood, especially the trauma of hospitalization and the birth of her sister when the patient was five years old. The separation difficulties that appeared in the transference were a repetition of these early times. The introjective defences within the transference indicated that these were the mechanisms which the patient utilized in childhood to dissipate the hate that had been brought about by loss. The patient's identification with the therapist was a new edition of the identification with the mother. This patient was never able to accept the hatred which she bore against her mother other than in an intellectual way.

The second phase of the therapy lasted for a very short time. At the beginning there was no special indication that the patient had altered. She tended to be silent and withdrawn, but her behaviour did not give rise to anxiety because it had appeared many times before. Gradually she became depressed in mood, and in a sense this development was unexpected, because things had seemed to be going well. A short time earlier she had started to go out with a man and seemed happy about it. Only later did she announce that the relationship had come to nothing. It was the disappointment that ushered in the second phase. She had chosen the man on the basis of narcissism. She overvalued intellect and her male friend was intelligent and well educated. Her choice was no doubt determined by transference.

Close scrutiny of the depressive outbreak showed that its onset coincided with a disagreement with her landlady. She was very angry with the woman, but no real cause could be found for her attitude. The patient's behaviour indicated that an aggravation of the mother relationship was already at work. Afterwards she became upset, saying that the therapist was angry with her and the landlady's behaviour was an indirect message from him announcing his annoyance.

In the next session the patient revealed that she had been experiencing auditory hallucinations for some time. The content of the hallucinations consisted of the therapist's voice speaking to her. Usually what he said was pleasant and reassuring. The voices indicated the closeness of the therapist. She believed that she had seen him walking beneath her window and she had also seen him at school. Associated with these ideas was a confused feeling of being mixed up, no longer an independent being, and of being unable to oppose the thoughts of those with whom she came in contact.

The transition from the second to the third phase was marked by the appearance of persecutory ideas. She accused the therapist of telling her landlady to annoy and upset her. She related a number of such activities, for which she blamed the therapist. The ventilation of these thoughts seemed to calm and reassure her. Now she revealed that she was no longer meeting her man friend.

During the next two months there seemed to be some signs of progress towards the gaining of insight into the irrational ideas. She acknowledged the guilt which had been stimulated by sexual interest in her man friend, and she appeared to be aware of the anger occasioned by her rejection. However, this favourable trend came to an end with the sudden appearance of a fully elaborated delusional complex. In great distress she related that the night before she had been forced to have sexual relations with the therapist—she had felt his body beside her. There were microphones and a television machine in the room, which transmitted all that was going on. When she experienced sexual feelings the therapist had sexual feelings. She felt as though she was a part of him. This was all arranged by the therapist's wife. The latter had obtained the help of her friends to injure and damage the patient and the therapist. They had made her think that she could have sexual relations with the therapist in order to incriminate her. She interpreted every environmental experience as related to this persecution. The patient was admitted to hospital at this time. Persecutory delusions and auditory hallucinations continued for a number of months, later to be accompanied by the reappearance of depressive symptoms.

In this case there was, during the pre-psychotic period, a partial withdrawal from the world of objects and a preoccupation with thoughts of the therapist. In metapsychological terms, a regression had affected object cathexes in such a way as to lead to a withdrawal of some of these cathexes from objects and their investment in phantasy and memory traces. Wishes came true — the therapist was with her, looking after her, and she could hear his voice. Guilt led to a fear of the landlady and her fear that she had displeased the therapist. Such an oedipal colouring of the manifest material is a common feature in psychotic states. Although this patient's narcissism had become pathological she had not abandoned her relationship with the object (the therapist). In this respect the clinical data were characteristic of phase one of Freud's model of psychoses — withdrawal (complete or partial) of object cathexes and a regression to a pathological narcissism.

The account of this patient's clinical history shows how hallucinatory experiences arose in relation to an object (the therapist). Many cases have been described in the psycho-analytic literature which demonstrate how wishful phantasies are transformed into hallucinatory experiences. Such phenomena may be found at the outset of many psychotic illnesses, and at this stage the patient still retains a strong contact with the object world. It would seem, therefore, that hallucinatory experiences of this type are quite compatible with the operation of object cathexes – that is, with the capacity for object relations. Such hallucinatory phenomena are not restitutional products – they do not have the aim of re-creating relationships with objects or of substituting a new reality for that of the environment as was seen to be the case with delusions. This approach raises the possibility of classifying hallucinations in functional terms. Hallucinations may be regarded either as restitutional in function or as a special form of object relationship.

Before proceeding to consider the further clinical history of hallucinations, it is necessary to consider other functions that may be performed by hallucinatory phenomena. It has frequently been noted that patients may hallucinate during the course of an interview. This observation provides good evidence for the theory that hallucinations are not 'endogenous' phenomena – arising from within the patient – but are in fact a response to a specific external stimulus. It has been known for a long time that there is a special category of auditory hallucinations that are provoked into activity by auditory stimuli. Examination of the specific stimulus usually reveals a symbolic or direct connection with an aspect of the patient's interpersonal relationships as they existed at the outset of the illness. In the following clinical illustration it is possible to observe the immediate stimulus for a hallucinatory experience.

HALLUCINATION AS THE MODE OF EXPRESSION OF LIBIDINAL AND DESTRUCTIVE WISHES

CASE 12. The patient was a married woman of thirty-five who was admitted to hospital because of neglect of her family duties, an increasing restlessness, grandiose delusions, passivity feelings, and auditory hallucinations. She talked freely but was frequently irritable, critical, and aggressive towards the interviewer, nurses, and other patients. Her hallucinatory experience took the form of the belief that other people spoke 'under her breath' – their lips did not move but she could hear them speaking. She also believed that everyone could read her thoughts. In turn, she knew what everyone else thought. The interview, excerpts from which are described below, followed a test situation in which the patients listened to a series of words – one of which was 'love' – over headphones. She spoke as follows.

Patient: 'I am just wondering why when I read everyone hears me.' (She took up a piece of paper and looked at it.) 'I am looking at this and you can hear what I am reading without saying it . . . just with the brain. You can do it . . .' *Interviewer:* 'Do you mean I can read your mind when you are reading?' *Patient:* 'Yes . . . you know what I am reading, dear . . . I wish I knew what that electrical treatment was for . . . is it for the brain?' *Interviewer:* 'What treatment?' *Patient:* 'Next door I was putting the lights into place . . . it's a space . . . it is to do with space value.' *Interviewer:* 'What do you mean?' *Patient:* 'In that place there . . . you press the buttons and put them into place . . . it's a moon . . . it's to do with space and speed and nerve in the brain. It is to do with the nerve and the brain and the speech . . . you don't care tuppence what I'm speaking about . . . when I am thinking everyone can hear what I'm thinking . . . it means you have nothing to yourself . . .'

After this the patient was silent for some time but then continued saying she had space-sickness. When asked in what way, she replied, 'Just the same as sea-sickness . . . you can get sea-sickness with that pipe you are smoking . . . and you can get fainting sickness but you can have the three in one.' *Interviewer:* 'What do you mean by the three in one?' *Patient:* 'You can be dead tired and collapse with the cigarette smoke and the nerve and the pipe and the three in one . . . What is the man next door — a radiograph or something . . . a scientist or something?' *Interviewer:* 'Why?' *Patient:* 'He's recording . . . he's not very good because he's too much on lights and things and wires and electricity . . . I don't care much for electricity. I don't like it very much . . . lights in the sky . . . you don't see them very often . . . but what's he got in there . . . because every time I used to look at the moon or something like that . . . got back on the television . . . they would speak under their breath like you do and they would tell me that I'm up there.' *Interviewer:* 'Am I speaking under my breath?' *Patient:* 'You do at times.' *Interviewer:* 'Did you hear me?' *Patient:* 'Yes.' *Interviewer:* 'When?' *Patient:* 'A wee while ago.' *Interviewer:* 'Where were you?' *Patient:* 'The same place as you.' *Interviewer:* 'Where was that?' *Patient:* 'Let me see now . . . between space value and dream and love life I should say . . . that's why you asked the question and I gave the answer . . . It was a wee while ago . . . you asked me a question and told me what to say . . . it was in here.' *Interviewer:* 'What did I say?' *Patient:* 'That I was clever or something . . . that's the main thing.' *Interviewer:* 'What else?' *Patient:* 'Love or something ... some person but it wasn't me. I don't stick to that way because I can't be bothered with it ... I would rather read a book ... I'm interested in space and in the Bible and in teaching children ... and electricity ... I should like to know why they are testing my head ... what is it for? ... from his point of view what is he doing? ... I don't know ... only I had a crack in my brain when I was wee ...'

She made some remark about the interviewer speaking under his breath and was asked why should he do that. She replied, 'I don't know ... it's feelings of your own you have ... sometimes you have to keep them to yourself ... I do ... the speaking under the breath is really speech ... only they are too frightened to put face value and say it out loud ... it's a wrong way ... why speak at all?' *Interviewer:* 'You mean I'm frightened to say what I'm thinking?' *Patient:* 'Yes ... You wouldn't say what you said ... under your breath to me ... because I might get up and hit you ... you wouldn't dare because you're a doctor and you love someone else ... you wouldn't dare.' *Interviewer:* 'To do what?' *Patient:* 'Whatever you're thinking ... unless it's got something to do with what I have been examined for.' *Interviewer:* 'What's that?' *Patient:* 'My head I should think.' *Interviewer:* 'What would I not dare tell you?' *Patient:* 'Talk about love life.' *Interviewer:* 'You mean that I was suggesting something sexual to you?' *Patient:* 'Yes ... yes it is, but it was just casual ... I think I'm teaching you.' *Interviewer:* 'Are you not talking about your own sexual thoughts?' *Patient:* 'Everyone has ... I'm a married woman ... it's natural ... but I can't be bothered with it very much ... I can't be bothered with it ...'

These clinical data demonstrate the manner in which an auditory hallucination appeared. The stimulus was the interviewing psychiatrist and the content was provided by the memory of a test word and the associations to which it gave rise. It was not surprising that the content of this woman's hallucinations should have had a libidinal nature because sexual (genital) conflicts were of importance in the precipitation of, and in forming the predisposition to, the illness. In this instance the hallucination was initiated by a libidinal drive cathexis but, unlike what occurs in the healthy or the psychoneurotic patient, the ideational content was not repressed but was subject to the process of topographic regression whereby it was converted into auditory percepts. This mechanism, which led to hallucination, had a defensive function in so far as the patient could disown responsibility for her sexual wishes.

Hallucinations, therefore, not only represent wishes related to objects – desired or lost – as fulfilled but also arise in order to banish from consciousness undesired wishes. In this respect the hallucinating patient differs radically from the psychoneurotic patient who employs more reliable and effective defence mechanisms. A woman patient who has started unconsciously to entertain libidinal phantasies about a psychiatrist, or any other kind of doctor for that matter, will banish such ideas from consciousness by the use of repression or projection. In the latter instance she may think that the physician is sexually interested in her. There are patients who will displace the transference phantasy to someone else and try to live it out with that particular person. This is the behaviour described as 'acting-out in the transference'. Hallucination, then, is an expression of a primitive type of defence against the drives – utilizing the mechanism of topographic regression.

Hallucinations with a hostile or destructive content arise in a similar fashion and are to be understood as the outcome of attempted defence against aggressive drives. This was the case in a woman of thirty-two who was in the habit of hallucinating during interviews. She became fearful, complaining that the voices were forcing her to smash the windows of the room. She would complain that she saw devils who tempted her. During one session she became angry with the interviewer because he said that he did not hear the voices or see the devils. She accused him of lying like the man who had seduced her in early adolescence. She freely admitted that one of the voices she heard was that of this man and thus was one of the devils. There had been many other sexual experiences at later times and therefore many other devils. The interviewer was a potential devil who would force her to sexual misdemeanours.

The patient could disown responsibility by blaming the devils' voices for her behaviour in just the same manner as she had blamed the men in the past for her promiscuity. Apart from this, however, she became hallucinated in interviews whenever aggressive urges were directed against the interviewer – she heard the voices telling her to break a window when he refused to prescribe extra sedation. In this case repudiated thoughts were converted into auditory percepts. Her fear of the interviewer was also displaced onto a fear of the voices. The auditory hallucinations could therefore be regarded as condensing both the patient's aggressive inclinations and her fear of retaliation.

The hallucinatory phenomena examined thus far have been seen to arise in relation to individuals who have or have had a significance for the patient. They either had the function of creating a wished-for relation-ship as actuality or they were the expression of a defensive conflict. Hallucinatory experiences serving these aims are to be found in clinical states of different kinds. Some clinicians might regard all cases manifesting auditory hallucinations as suffering from schizophrenia, whereas others might consider some as non-schizophrenic psychoses – diagnosing the conditions as atypical manic-depressive psychosis or as hysterical psychosis. This failure to agree on a diagnosis indicates how difficult it is to obtain reliable assessments of a clinical state when the diagnosis is based solely upon clinical phenomena that are examined in isolation. The psycho-analytic approach suggests that an identical mechanism may operate in different clinical states, thus leading to similar types of clinical manifestation.

It was suggested earlier that the hallucinatory data described so far are not to be regarded as the outcome of measures directed to regaining contact with the world of objects, because such phenomena are associ-ated with a residual capacity to make relationships. Object cathexes are still operating. These patients had either brought to life a wish phantasy or defended themselves against the intrusion of unwelcome urges into consciousness.

It is important to differentiate between hallucinations whose content consists of the realization of a wished-for relationship and those in which the content consists of the return of a lost relationship. A number of psycho-analytical authors (Havens, 1962; Modell, 1958) have de-monstrated clinically that hallucinatory voices represent memories – perhaps in a distorted form – of relationships which were once of great emotional significance to the patient. Havens (1962) has proposed that hallucinations occur in order to satisfy needs for specific objects, which are usually unattainable in reality.

In the following case a clinical illustration is presented in which the hallucinatory experience did not consist of an attempt to build up a substitute world through delusional complexes but was an attempt to restore a lost object relationship.

HALLUCINATION AS A COMPENSATION FOR OBJECT LOSS

CASE 13. The patient was a single woman of twenty-seven who complained that a man whom she had previously admired was reading her mind and talking to her. This caused her great distress. She said that she heard his voice in her head. She had never had any close relationship with him, but from the age of sixteen had been in love with him. She frankly admitted that she used to think constantly about him, dream about him, and enjoy erotic phantasies.

She had heard his voice for about a year before she consulted a doctor. During that time it was a pleasurable experience. In this respect, and at this phase of the illness, the patient's hallucinations were identical with those in the first case reported above. In the years between sixteen and twenty-three she firmly believed that she and her admired friend would come together. The man was forty-two and unmarried. When she was twenty-three she heard from friends that there was some suspicion that he was a homosexual. From this time on she came to believe that he was reading her thoughts and what he said was disturbing and unpleasant. The hallucinatory experience had continued for three years. She had twice been in hospital, where she was treated with electro-shock therapy and tranquillizers. These treatments had led to a brief remission of symptoms.

The patient's capacity to communicate was in no way impaired and she was willing to discuss her experiences. She said that the man knew everything she was thinking and she read his mind also. She could hear more than once voice — often it seemed the man was quarrelling with someone else. She believed that he was not working and at times a voice said that he would have to go into hospital because he was mentally ill. There were times when the voice told lies and she would seem to be involved in a quarrel with it. After a number of interviews she said that the man was also being seen by a doctor. She believed that whatever happened to her was also happening to him. She saw no connection between herself and the activities of the phantasy object, even at a later stage when she expressed the belief that the man was in the same hospital as herself.

She told the interviewer that he did not believe what she told him. This projection of her own insight continued throughout the clinical contact. She complained bitterly that she was ill mentally. By this she meant that she could not concentrate or remember anything because the voice was interfering with her mental activity. She attributed aspects of her cognition to the delusional object in the same manner as Modell (1958) described in his patients. She would forget where her cigarettes were and, after she had looked everywhere for them, a voice would say, 'They are in your locker', and that is where she would find them. Similarly, she attributed many of her own thoughts to the voice.

In spite of an unwillingness to communicate, she did reveal the phantasy (delusional) that the man was in the hospital. She was always expecting to meet him. Soon after this she told the interviewer that he was seeing the man before coming to see her. Then she announced that it was her father who was reading her mind and speaking to her, although it was through the man's voice. She became acutely upset. She did not know what to believe and for the most part she would refuse to report what the voice was saying but mutter, 'It's all lies.'

Her distress increased – she believed the man was in the ward above the one in which she was resident. She could hear his footsteps upstairs whenever she walked up and down. She would ask, 'What's going on?' but would not express herself further. Everything that had happened in the ward was of significance. Every noise was meaningful – she looked for microphones in the consulting-room and was constantly searching for the man. One day she was convinced she had seen him at the window. Eventually, the interviewer was reading her mind. She oscillated between the belief that the interviewer knew everything that was happening or that he did not believe that she heard a voice at all.

In this case of hallucinatory psychosis the mechanisms underlying the symptoms could be easily discerned. At the outset of the illness the phantasies of the admired man reached hallucinatory intensity, probably during the period before sleep or while day-dreaming. After the realization of the inevitable disappointment, the object was introjected into the ego and became a part of it. This was to be seen, first, in the patient's inability to discriminate her own activity from that of the internalized object and, second, in her attributing her cognitive functions to it. The internalization can be regarded as a compensatory process, in the sense that the ensuing symptoms represent the patient's restoration of the lost object.

The withdrawal and loss of interest in real objects were demonstrated in her attitude and behaviour towards the interviewer. She was indifferent to him and uninfluenced by his comments or interpretations. She was taken up entirely with the internalized object, which was oedipal in nature. Gradually the interviewer was drawn into the delusional complex but only in so far as she could not imagine that he was not in contact with the internalized object.

Throughout the clinical material there ran an exaggerated egocentrism in which the self was the centre of environmental events. These data can be understood as being due to an ego regression that reduced cognition to that developmental level where thinking and perceiving are tied to the current environmental context and where there is no abstraction from it. Thus everything relates to the self and is judged according to this standard. The libidinal drives were initially instrumental in awakening the phantasy memories. These memories were later experienced as auditory percepts. It is quite likely that the conversion of feeling from love to hate resulted from rage against the disappointing object. A similar sequence of events has been reported by Cameron (1961). In the case described here the patient had no hesitation is saying how much she hated the persecutor and that she would like to murder him.

The cases reported show that auditory hallucinations can arise, first, as a response to an interpersonal contact and, second, as a means whereby the patient restores a lost object relationship. Hatred arising from disappointment can lead to the formerly loved object being converted into a persecutor, as was clear in the last example. There is an argument, therefore, for believing that hallucinatory phenomena have different functions, even though they may have a common origin in a topographic regression.

A CLASSIFICATION OF HALLUCINATIONS

Hallucinations can be classified into two distinct categories. First, there are those which are closely bound to real objects and where the clinical state is not characterized by an extreme state of withdrawal. It follows that in such cases the patient may still be capable of transference if offered the opportunity of a therapeutic relationship. The deciding factor in this respect will be how far the object cathexes have been internalized and invested in the hallucinatory object. In the last case quoted the investment was considerable. The patient was able to participate in a treatment relationship, but her object cathexes never reached the therapist for they were totally bound up with the internalized object. In other types of hallucinatory psychosis where the hallucination expresses an underlying defensive conflict, the patient can often make adequate transferences that enable an analysis of the hallucinatory phenomena to be undertaken.

The second category of hallucinations are those which are solely concerned with the construction of a new psychic reality. Clinical experience favours the view that the first hallucinatory experiences, which characterize psychotic states that proceed to chronicity and deterioration of personality (dementia praecox), are of a similar type to the first category. In these malignant states the hallucinatory phenomena do not remain unaltered in their content and are accompanied by indications of an extensive withdrawal from object relationships. Object cathexes not only are lost but also alter their quality in the direction of instinctualization (deneutralization). At the outset of these serious illnesses the contents of the hallucinations generally comprise wished-for and/or lost object relations. They may also signify the presence of a defensive conflict. As the condition progresses, it becomes apparent that the hallucinations tend to become an integral aspect of a new psychic reality which the patient substitutes for the reality of the environment, as in the case of delusions. Every environmental experience is altered to accord with what has been psychically constructed. Although the hallucinatory phenomena can, in the same way as the delusions, be traced back to origins in relationships that once existed, they have now acquired an autonomy, an independence from their original source. In this respect they differ from the first category of hallucinations, which always remain tied to environmental objects.

It is well known that in chronic schizophrenic states hallucinations may take different forms and affect any of the sensory modalities. At times the hallucinations can be recognized as resulting from environmental stimuli, but at other times it is difficult to account for the stimulus and for the content. In Case 8 (Chapter 5) the patient received instructions from the hallucinatory schoolmaster and the content of the hallucinations could be understood as an externalization of the patient's wishes, attitudes, and judgements. In this respect the hallucinatory experiences were a means of environmental adjustment. The presence of the hallucinatory voice gave the patient a sense of security. On one occasion when the voice disappeared for two or three days she was acutely anxious. Even in the most chronic case, however, if the patient is willing to discuss his experiences, it is often possible to discover the stimulus for them and the reason for their content. Although the hallucinations of chronic patients achieve an autonomy and thus serve a restitutional function, they are no less sensitive to arousal by stimuli arising from current relationships. In a case now to be described, the hallucinations, which were primarily restitutional in nature, were easily activated by external stimulation. In contrast to the cases described in earlier sections of this chapter, this patient's hallucinations were not related to one particular individual. They were activated by doctors, patients, and nurses. It was thus possible to observe the immediate stimulus for these hallucinatory experiences and to note a similar mechanism to that which occurs in non-schizophrenic psychoses.

HALLUCINATIONS AS THE EXPRESSION OF RESTITUTION AND ADAPTATION

CASE 14. The patient was a married woman of forty who had been hospitalized for a period of nine years. Her illness had started suddenly. She had been living with her husband in Persia until political upheavals led to the evacuation of the families of British employees. When the patient and her husband resumed life together she began to accuse him of infidelity. There was some reality in these reproaches and eventually the husband left her for another woman. It was reported that she had become increasingly uninterested in and neglectful of her home and children. On admission to hospital she continued to criticize her husband and complained of feeling vaguely unwell. Apart from this there was no obvious psychotic symptomatology. Gradually, evidence of thought disorder, hallucinatory experience, and inappropriate affect were obtained. Insulin coma treatment had no effect upon her condition.

The patient was greatly troubled by her sexual feelings. She attempted to deal with these feelings by projection. She accused other patients, nurses, and doctors of making her dirty. A typical statement was as follows.

Patient: 'That's not me' (looking at herself in the mirror). 'They put me inside people while I am sitting on a chair. That's not me . . . dirty face, dirty teeth, dirty brain, dirty thoughts. Animals take you, that's what they do.' When she was asked what she meant by this, she replied, 'They put me in the televison. A big crocodile took a man in the swamp (this was a reference to a film on the television the day before) . . . it took me . . . The face said it was taking me even although I was sitting. I had a bad night last night but I went to sleep with someone else's head. That's what they want to do with me . . . I don't like Miss X (another patient) she puts dirty thoughts in my mind. She rams in Eastern thoughts and things that appear on the television. They can see everything that goes on in me. I'm a fool. I go on sitting. I don't want to be taken sexually because I'm not made right. It's a trick of the mind, I can't take, it's only afterwards I know.' By the expression 'take' she meant the arousal of a genital sensation akin to vaginal penetration.

During a restless phase she would march up and down the ward shouting abuse at patients and staff. She would say, 'They are dirty.' On one occasion she came to a halt beside a picture. She shouted at the picture, 'You are dirty, getting inside me.' She lifted the picture from the wall and smashed it on the floor. She became afraid of what she had done and said, 'I won't take the responsibility of that, it was you. The doctor is to blame, glass is a mere detail . . . I will not be responsible they are playing different parts, I'm never me.' When the incident was discussed with her later, she appeared to be pleased with herself and said, 'I like the man in the picture – I liked his appearance.' She told the interviewer that voices told her to lie down on a couch and put a pillow under her hips. This was the position she adopted in intercourse with her husband. Frequently these auditory hallucinations led to outbursts of rage, and here she projected her guilt onto some other patients in the ward. These libidinal outbursts were as frequently homosexual as heterosexual in their origins. The heterosexual tendencies could be traced to her attachment to the ward doctor. It was libidinal arousal from this source which generated the command to lie down with a pillow under her hips.

This patient also complained of visual hallucinations. She would accuse other patients of throwing her husband and children at her. When she was asked to explain what she meant by this, she said that the other patients were throwing pictures of her husband and children. She did not want to see them because it was too painful. She explained that she had not seen them for many years and the memory of them made her extremely unhappy. It can by hypothesized that the visual hallucinations were the result of wishes to be with her family once again. The cathexes underlying these wishes awakened memories which were experienced as visual percepts. The patient denied their origin in herself and projected them because of their painful quality. She did not wish to be reminded of the name of her husband or the names of her children. Her only defence against mental pain was outbursts of rage.

DISCUSSION AND SUMMARY

Throughout this chapter little attention has been given to the superego aspects of hallucinatory phenomena. It is the externalization and the fragmentation of the superego which leads to the fear of the hallucinations and to their persecutory content. Without these superego influences hallucinations would be either pleasurable, informative or instructing.

Modell (1958) has pointed out that it is erroneous to attribute all hallucinatory experience to superego activity, because all hallucinations are not persecutory in content. Much hallucinatory activity, as in many of the cases described here, arises from the ego — that is from attitudes, memories, and judgements which are subsequently ascribed to the voices. In patients of this kind there is often no evidence of persecutory content. It is true, nevertheless, that the complexity of hallucinatory content results from wishes that give rise to anxiety and guilt and it is this which leads to the frightening experiences. The recollection of unwanted memories can lead to mental pain and when these memories return as percepts the same pain is experienced, although now attributed to the activity of the persecutor. Anxiety, guilt, and depressive affects can arise as a reaction to the hallucinated content.

It is a common practice to categorize hallucinations in terms of the modality concerned and in accordance with the content. The view has been advanced here that there is clinical justification for a more fundamental categorization. According to this view, hallucinations can be divided into two groups depending upon the function of the hallucination. In the first category the hallucinatory experiences are related to specific objects, and may symbolize the realization of a wish or replace a lost relationship. They may also have a defensive function. In such instances the hallucination can represent a repudiated wish or retribution for the wish or both. This type of hallucination does not form part of a 'complex' that substitutes for relationships in the world of reality.

The second category of hallucination comprises those phenomena which have become part of an attempt to create a new reality. They participate in providing a new substitute for the reality which has been lost as a consequence of the disease process. The mechanism underlying both categories of hallucinations is identical — the mechanism of topographic regression. The hallucinations obtain their energy from cathexes originally directed towards significant objects. In the second category the hallucinations detach themselves from their original objects and as the disease progresses displace themselves to real or phantasy objects of childhood or adolescence. When the illness is fully established the hallucinations appear to be completely isolated from objects. However, clinical contact with such patients shows (as in the last case quoted) that hallucinatory experience can arise once again, thus demonstrating the mode of origin and the basic mechanism underlying the clinical phenomena.

This approach to the understanding of hallucinations is based upon the psycho-analytic theory of object relationships. According to this view, two categories of hallucination can be delineated, which in fact represent extremes of a range. At one end are the hallucinatory states where there is little loss of the object-relationship capacity – object cathexes still operate. At the other end of the scale are those patients in whom the hallucinations (and delusions) completely consume what remains of their disorganized and deneutralized object cathexes. Contact with the world of objects is at a minimum. Between these extremes are varying degrees of object-relationship capacity and hallucinatory phenomena of appropriate type.

This psycho-analytically based categorization does away with the necessity of finding hallucinations that are specific in form and content for different forms of psychotic state. According to psycho-analytic theory, hallucinatory experiences may occur in any abnormal mental state because of the inherent potential in every human being for topographic regression. It also lays stress on the fact that hallucinatory phenomena must not be studied in isolation but must be examined in their relationship to the totality of mental function and in particular to the capacity for object relationships.

CHAPTER 7

The Reaction of Patients to an Experimental Situation

Psycho-analysis can play an important role in assessing the significance of the responses of psychotic patients to experimental situations. Reference was made in the introductory chapter to the so-called 'attitude' variable (Shakow, 1962), which probably accounts for a great deal of the variation in results produced in test situations by patients suffering from psychosis. Psycho-analysis, concentrating as it does on the conative aspects of mental function, is in a position to offer insights into the factors that constitute the 'attitude' variable. The present chapter will begin with some brief comments upon those aspects of psycho-analytic theory which bear upon this topic. These will be followed by a detailed account of the reactions of some patients who were presented with a simple task.

The data presented by the patients show how test situations can activate phantasies and become the focus for the displacement of psychic reactions. Psychotic patients are especially informative in this respect because their phantasies really become conscious, possibly as a consequence of the predominance of psychic reality. These patients contrast vividly with non-psychotic patients, whose psychic reality is hidden as a result of effective defence (repression) only to appear indirectly in dreams, in subtle allusions, or in altered bodily function.

PSYCHO-ANALYTIC ASPECTS OF EXPERIMENTATION

In Chapter 2 an account was given of the psycho-analytic theory (Rosenfeld, 1952; Bion, 1957) which postulates that the phenomena that may be noted during consecutive interviews with psychotic patients are to be regarded as an expression of transferences from the earliest infantile period. From the moment the patient meets the clinician, his utterances and behaviour reflect a particular aspect of his object-relationship patterns. When these data appear within the context of the patient-physician situation, they are described as transference psychosis. The hypothesis of a psychotic transference rests upon the theory (see Chapter 2) that the infant passes through a developmental phase which is psychotic in form and content (persecutory and melancholic). It follows from this theory that an experimental situation in which the patient is placed that is closely associated with clinical interviews will be influenced by these psychotic transferences. In addition, the experimenter and his apparatus will provoke further psychotic transferences on their own account.

The hypothesis is a valuable one because it alerts the investigator to the possibility of transferred and direct reactions to the experimental situation. The view has already been expressed (see Chapter 3) that psychotic transference phenomena are not 'genuine' transferences, but this is irrelevant at this point. If the patient under investigation suffered from a psychoneurosis and was simultaneously undergoing psychoanalytic therapy, then displaced reactions from the therapy to the experiment would be expected and would occur. In this instance, the displaced reactions would be aspects of a repetitive pattern of childhood responses activated by the therapy itself (transference neurosis). Fisher (1956) has shown, in the course of his tachistoscopic experiments with patients suffering from various kinds of neurotic disorder, that the response to the experiment is frequently determined by transference reactions.

The theory of psychotic transference would lead an investigator to suspect that in some cases the patient would show an aggravation of symptoms and poor performance on a task demanding a high level of cognitive functioning. This would follow in the case of a withdrawn, negativistic patient, because the experiment and the investigator would become the recipient of the patient's feared destructiveness as well as the repudiated parts of his ego (projective identification). At the same time, introjection of the projected hate and ego parts would lead to further withdrawal and fragmentation of cognition (see Chapter 2).

The theoretical differences that exist between the theory of psychotic transference and classical psycho-analytic theory are of less importance in the present context than recognition of the fact that psychotic patients, and schizophrenic patients in particular, will react to experimental situations with various kinds of responses generated by endopsychic 'complexes'. According to the classical psycho-analytic theory of psychosis, the response of a patient subjected to an experimental procedure will depend upon the extent to which the psychotic disorder has affected the ego organization and the instinctual base of object relations. If regression of object-libidinal cathexes has proceeded to a pathological narcissistic state or to a hypothesized autoerotic stage, then the patient will be incapable of 'genuine' transference (see Chapter 5).

Where there is an extensive disorganization of object cathexes, transference will not take place to the physician nor will it pass over to the experimental situation. The delusions and hallucinations, which are regarded in the classical theory as restitutional products, may attach themselves to the physician in the course of the detailed clinical study although, according to this view, these phenomena are not to be regarded as 'genuine' transferences (see Chapter 3). In patients of this kind, the cathexes that would be available for object relationships are taken up in the delusions. Such objects as appear in the delusions are often a distorted representation of childhood memories and phantasies. It follows from the classical theory that a patient may respond quite adequately to an experimental situation because it has no special significance for him. On the other hand, he may refuse to co-operate if the experiment becomes linked with his delusional ideation.

The classical theory sets out to explain why the symptomatology in the schizophrenias may vary in extent and form and why the patient may still retain some capacity for object relations. It is suggested that, resulting from the fact that the totality of mental functioning is not involved by the disease process, a residual capacity for normal mental activity remains. The possibility of using psycho-analysis as a means of 'information retrieval' (Kety, 1961) will depend, therefore, upon the extent of these 'non-psychotic residues' (Davie & Freeman, 1961). During the analytic treatment or study of schizophrenic and paranoid patients, phenomena appear that are similar to those encountered during phases of transference resistance in the psycho-analysis of the neuroses (see Chapter 3). This type of data may disappear to be replaced by negativism, withdrawal, misidentifications, the emergence of persecutory delusions which are attached to the person of the clinician. During periods when transference capacities reappear with the repetition of childhood conflicts and anxieties, there is every chance that they will spread over and influence the patient's behaviour in the experimental situation.

The psycho-analytic approach alerts the investigator to the possibility that the psychotic patient will react to the experimental situation independently of its content, particularly if it is initiated during a period of intensive clinical study. Most acute reactions to experimental situations are provided by two categories of patient: first, those who incorporate the experiment into their persecutory delusions and, second, those with a residual transference capacity and relatively intact ego functioning. It is patients of the second kind who displace into the experimental setting the transference phantasies which originate in the patient-clinician relationship. Reactions of both types can occur in the same patient at different periods of the illness.

Patients' reactions must be given serious attention because of the rapid growth of experimental psychiatry. Very often the techniques employed only consist of asking the patient to co-operate in the completion of a test which has been designed to measure the performance of a specific cognitive function or to identify and/or quantify a particular character trait. At other times the investigations are elaborate and complex. The majority of investigations are conducted with large numbers of patients and the results are compared with those obtained from control groups matched for age, sex, intelligence, and social class.

It is extremely difficult to isolate and identify the causes of individual reactions to the majority of experimental studies. This is a serious problem, because the results obtained from current studies are only applicable to groups of patients or subjects. They do not give much information about the individual patient. This means that the results of tests or experiments do not provide information that the clinician can utilize for diagnosis or prognosis.

At the beginning of the chapter reference was made to the fact that the conditions operating in many psychoses lead to phantasy reactions that are unconscious in the healthy or the psychoneurotic individual. In the following accounts of the responses of patients suffering from psychoses, it is possible to note the extent and influence of such phantasy reactions. In each case the patient had been seen daily for several weeks before being subjected to a simple test of attention. The test to which the patient had to attend consisted of his having to press a key when a light appeared before him. There were two lights flashing alternately and two keys which had to be pressed when the appropriate light appeared.

CLINICAL ILLUSTRATIONS

The Experiment as a Mental Stimulus

CASE 15. The patient was a single man of twenty who said that the souls of dead relatives and the soul of John the Baptist kept talking to him. He believed that Christ had entered his body to render him fit for heaven. The penetration of his body had taken place when he was lying on his bed at home. Jesus lay on top of him and his spirit entered the patient's body. Jesus was then re-formed in the patient's body, the result being that the patient could not discriminate between those parts of his body which were his and those which were Christ's. The main persecutor — John the Baptist — wanted Christ to remain imprisoned in the patient's body so that he could impersonate Christ in heaven. The patient felt that the only way to liberate Christ was to kill himself. John the Baptist and the other spirits were able to alter his bodily and mental state. They would threaten, insult, or bribe him. After an interview the voices said, 'If you don't mention we're haunting you, you will get your job back at the Co-op.'

Much of the hallucinatory content during the interviews consisted of the patient's unspoken reaction to the daily sessions. He would report as follows: 'The spirits told me the doctors are puzzled by the whole thing', or 'You should ask the doctor what he is going to do', or 'Dr F doesn't believe God is in you.' Though the patient spoke in a rational and coherent manner, he employed a number of special words (neologisms) which were related to his delusional preoccupations. Some of these words filtered through from Jesus and they might appear in the content of his hallucinations. This content and the activity of the persecutors provided excellent information regarding the patient's attitude to the interviews and the interviewer. On one occasion he complained after leaving a session, that the spirits had given him a headache. They were 'watering' his brain as he put it. Although he denied that he was afraid of the interviewer, the fear was obvious in the 'brainwashing' allusion.

The interviews became an important stimulus for reactions within the patient, and they constantly appeared in his hallucinations, as described above. They also took the form of bodily responses usually attributed to the action of the spirits. The antithesis which existed between the patient's conscious and pre- (? un-)conscious attitudes towards the interviewer was illustrated by his statement, 'They are saying to me that you (the interviewer) said I'm a wee imbecile.' This was said a few seconds after he had reported that he found the meetings helpful in resisting the influence of the spirits. The hallucinatory voices (the souls) condensed the patient's own aggressive drives and the fear of retaliation for this aggression. The retribution which he feared would be exacted by the souls was fused in the patient's mind with the interviewer. This awareness of the interviewer-soul condensation helped to clarify the patient's reaction to the test situation.

As might have been expected, the patient attributed his curiosity about the tests and his thoughts about the motives behind them to the souls. The souls told him he was keeping secrets from them. They looked forward to the interviews so that they could hear what he was thinking. Here the equation souls = interviewer was clear enough. He said the souls laughed throughout the test, saying it was ridiculous to submit Father to a test of sanity.

The following verbatim statement, recorded after a test session, demonstrated the way in which the test became identified with the spirits and activated his delusional phantasies.

'There is nothing else I can really tell you about it all . . . they have watered it but they don't know whether they have cleaned out my head . . . my head might have been tired and the water they had been using might have wakened up my head and if he [Jesus] still won't talk to me it may be my head they have wakened up but they haven't harmed Jesus . . . they water to read the head and I say curiosity killed the cat and I'm not curious . . . it may be my head they have wakened up through water . . . that is what baffles them and what baffles me too . . . they tried to have me read the head and I say curiosity killed the cat and I'm not curious to know what's inside my head, I'm not curious about that too . . . but they are.'

When it was suggested that he was afraid that the test would reveal something he wanted to hide, he replied, 'No I don't know what they (the souls) think of all this. I think of Mr G [the experimenter] sometimes and his machine. I think when I operate the machine that I do it quite well . . . I know I do it quite well myself but they still talk but I can manage to look and work the machine and listen to them at the same time. I think this is what Mr G means – are there really spirits bothering him? . . . he thinks we'll see how his concentration is on the blue and red signals, to see how he makes out with them . . . of course it can't read my mind . . . I don't think you doctors can read what's in my mind . . . I don't think anyone could do that . . . it's impossible for anyone to do so . . . but they still talk and they said that the doctors think I'm quite well enough to work . . . I heard the spirits say that Dr F thinks you can do a job of work, that's what they said to me . . . that you were thinking I could do a job of work . . . You see they were just laughing to themselves, but I was more interested in the signals . . . they had taken my mind from them but they still talk . . . they take my mind from them so that I can concentrate on you, Dr F or Mr G, and whatever he has to do with his machine I can concentrate and work it.'

The above excerpt shows how this patient reacted to the test situation. He was able to perform quite well in spite of the hallucinatory experiences. In his case the psychical complexes did not have a disrupting effect upon performance. It was as if the test situation was just another environmental situation which was assimilated and recast in terms of the current psychic reality.

The Experimenter as a Transference Object

CASE 16. The patient was a single woman of nineteen who was admitted to hospital because of disturbed behaviour, hallucinatory experiences, and fleeting persecutory ideas. When she was examined by the admitting doctor (a woman) her speech content was disordered. She could not sustain a theme and would wander to irrelevant subjects. The following is a verbatim statement at the time of admission: 'You have the same eyes (referring to the doctor), the same mouth, the same nose . . . what age are you? . . . are you my mother . . . are you any relation to me? . . . I fell when I was very young and damaged my head . . . you gave me one good eye . . . I was trying to get some breath and you were breathing in and out for me . . . ' She giggled inappropriately and was distractable. She misidentified people, said she had diabetes and that her eye was twisted.

The young woman was a student nurse at an ophthalmic hospital. At the first interview after admission she said that she was getting married that day to a patient whom she had nursed in the eye hospital. He had been operated upon for a left strabismus. She had heard his voice and believed that she was pregnant. At the next interview she complained of blurred vision and demanded dark glasses. Her identification with the phantasied lover was complete. His voice was with her all the time. She misidentified nurses and patients. She was distractable, reacting readily to extraneous stimuli.

She asked the interviewer if he heard the voices saying she was pregnant. She complained of abdominal pain and transient persecutory ideas. She had no difficulty in communicating, even although the

K

content of her speech was disconnected. She showed a tendency to identify with the interviewer, saying, 'I'm falling asleep in the arm-chair', when he had yawned and felt drowsy. She was tested on four successive days after having been seen daily for a number of weeks. Her first comment was to complain of a headache and say that she had parts of other people's bodies in her. She complained than an electrical current was being passed through her bed and that the nurses were trying to make her commit suicide.

She made few references to the test beyond saying that it was to see if she had cancer. It was also to save her mother's life. After the second test she told the interviewer that she was a doctor and repeated that the test was to save her mother's life: 'To save my mother's life, my sister's life, there is radium in the light . . . it hits the heart . . . when you press the light gently . . . I am quick tempered . . . it makes you go to sleep . . . I asked the night nurse for a cup of milk . . . it's to see if I'm a drug addict . . . ' She continued in this chaotic fashion in the two following interviews, successively identifying the test apparatus as a machine necessary for open-heart surgery: ' . . . the test proves you can heal your own heart . . . ' Throughout these interviews she kept referring to a friend called Margaret Love – but it was possible that the name 'Love' had been provoked by the word 'love' heard over the earphones. She also insisted that the women in the ward were prostitutes.

After the fourth testing session the word 'love' was even more to the fore in her comments: ' . . . I fell from my mother's womb . . . she went from country to country . . . two parts were affected . . . the heart and reproductive organs – I cannot bear children and I love everybody . . . ' Back in the ward she believed something dangerous was going on. She described a machine identical with the test apparatus which was hidden in the ward and could induce sexual feelings in her. She felt afraid.

She accused a woman doctor to whom she had been speaking of trying to turn her into a prostitute. This datum was clarified by the declaration that she had fallen in love with the psychologist who had administered the test. She spoke as follows.

Patient: ' . . . I'm a doctor . . . I'll tell you . . . I fell in love for the first time today.' *Interviewer:* 'Who with?' *Patient:* ' . . . the doctor who gives you all the tests. He wore a tartan tie; left, right, and centre (a reference to the lateral movement of the lights) to see your brain is working all right – what are you trying to do? Drown me . . . I need his mind and he needs mine. We're made for each other . . . good company sticks together . . . but he had a short life and so did I; left, right, and centre. I love you, simple . . . long engagement . . . that's what a test pilot does every night.'

This young woman was unable to perform the test situation in a satisfactory manner. She was constantly distracted, possibly by phantasies about the psychologist. This sexualization was identical with the earlier one when she nursed in the eye hospital. The libidinal urges provoked anxiety and her utterances revealed the persecutory phantasies that were activated – being punished by electricity, becoming a prostitute, and becoming ill. At other times she defended herself against these wishes by projection. She blamed the machine, the test apparatus, or the doctor for inducing sexual feeling, or she accused her mother or the patients (who were often condensed) of being prostitutes. She hallucinated the psychologist's voice in just the same way as she had heard her own patient's voice. In this case phantasies expressed in fragmentary fashion were stimulated by the experimental apparatus and the experimenter himself.

The Experimental Situation as a Vehicle for 'Acting-out in the Transference'

CASE 17. The third reaction to be described is taken from the fifty-year-old woman patient whose case was described in Chapter 3. There details were given of the first eight weeks of the interview material. This demonstrated how the patient sexualized the relationship with the interviewer. The sexualization appeared to be related to a seduction at puberty. However, data obtained later, and not reported in Chapter 3, revealed that just prior to the onset of her illness she had had a liaison with her son's friend. This patient's readiness for libidinal arousal led to the development of phantasies, expectations, and fears in relation to the interviewer. She entertained pregnancy phantasies which were expressed in a delusional manner. References were made to this in the first eight weeks when she talked about being interfered with sexually in the hospital.

The sexualization of the interview situation led to intense resistances on the patient's part. She was hostile, unco-operative, tantalizing, on the one hand, and depressed, self-critical, and dejected, on the other. Outbursts of rage would, as a result of introjection, be converted into bouts of self-criticism and suicidal thoughts. She had little capacity for dealing with disappointment and its effects. Associated with this content were narcissistic phenomena consisting of the belief that the interviewer was omnipotent, controlled her mind, and forced her to his will. These data was interpreted (not to the patient) as the unconscious wish and fear of genital union with the interviewer — sadistically represented.

When the patient entered the test situation after nearly four months of daily interviews, she did so preoccupied with sadistic transference phantasies. These phantasies, denied expression through verbalization, sought out objects through which they might find an outlet. In addition, the anxiety and guilt stimulated by the phantasies provided a further source of stress. Her initial reaction to the test was motivated by her guilt. She accused the interviewer of wanting to 'brainwash' her and find out things against her will. The sadistic preoccupations emerged first in accusations against the interviewer of brutality and of torturing her by the test. She meant by this that the red light which flashed during the test had been put there to remind her of destructive activities which she had in fact initiated against her husband in the past.

It was, however, in the second series of test sessions that the patient unconsciously exploited the test apparatus as a means whereby the sadistic sexual phantasies could find an actual expression — an 'acting out' of the transference neurosis which had developed in the interview situation. She admitted, after interpretation, that she wanted to smash the apparatus. She justified this wish on the ground that the apparatus had reminded her of machinery which had mutilated a neighbour's son. At the second test of the series she threw the headphones to the ground, and in the following interview insisted that the apparatus was a means of dragging out her sexual thoughts about the interviewer.

In this case the test apparatus was sexualized and, as a consequence of the patient's own sadism, came to represent by displacement and projection the sexually damaging interviewer. On a more primitive level it possibly symbolized the destructive penis.

This woman's performance was very poor in all the tests in spite of the fact that there was no clinical evidence of cognitive disorganization. Apart from her delusional ideas, she could converse rationally and attend to tasks. There could be little doubt that her poor performance was caused by the endopsychic factors described above.

The Experiment as a Stimulus for New Delusional Content

CASE 18. The patient was a single man of thirty-two who complained that a number of unknown, evil people interfered with his bodily and mental activities by means of rays. The rays could induce painful and sexual sensations. The persecutors wanted to use his brains for thinking. He was unable to be angry because he could not find anyone to be angry with. He was distressed, fearing that his heart might be affected by the rays. The rays paralysed his movements — if he wanted to raise his arm a ray would be fired at his head and paralyse the movement. He was unable to put a cigarette in his mouth if the rays were employed against him.

At the outset of the clinical contact he expressed himself as pleased because he disliked what he believed to be the effect of the phenothiazine drugs. This medication had been discontinued when the interviews began. After a week his attitude to the meetings altered. His fears of the effects of the meetings — they might be 'overpowering' — came very close to his description of the interference by the rays. It looked as if the patient imposed the role of persecutor upon the interviewer. The statement of this fear was followed by frequent silences during the interviews and by protestations that he had nothing more to say.

He expressed a dislike for the meetings, saying that coming daily gave him a feeling of being trapped. The rays began to operate during the sessions. Their effect was to block his awareness of what the interviewer said. The patient was now having recourse to his delusional preoccupation to express his resistance to the interview situation. He could disclaim responsibility for this resistance, since everything was out of his control. Anxiety regarding the direction his thoughts might take during the interviews led to the production of abnormal experiences.

As the interviews continued, the effect of the rays increased. He complained that he was unable to concentrate or attend. He reported that during one or two sessions the effect of the rays was less and this led to an improvement in his attitude to the interviewer. This improvement may have been due to the fact that he could now remain silent in the meetings without the interviewer pressing him to reveal his thoughts. After some further meetings he was able to speak about the rays and give more details about them. For the next weeks he either was silent or repetitiously referred to the persecution by the rays. His defence was impenetrable — nothing emerged about his current life or about his past. A contact with the observer was possible as long as his fears could be attributed to the rays and not to the interviewer or to his own thoughts.

The effect of the first test session was to alter his description of the manner in which the rays entered his body. He said that, though the rays came over all his body, they were now concentrated on two spots on the frontal region of the head. His emphasis on the concentration of rays into two beams may have been due to his awareness of the two lights of the test apparatus. In the interval between the first and second test sessions no change was to be observed. He avoided responsibility for angry words against another patient by blaming the rays. He apologized to this patient, explaining that the rays had raised his arm and made him curse. When the interviewer asked him why this happened, he showed his hostility and contempt by saying, 'I leave that to fools — thinking is a lot of nonsense.' Relating his thoughts was what he had been asked to do by the interviewer from the start of the meetings. He disagreed when the interviewer pointed to his latent hostility. He thought this nonsense. Nevertheless his comment and his refusal to acknowledge its real purpose (expression of anger against the interviewer), paralleled his cursing the other patient and the form of his apology.

The conflict between the omnipotent destructiveness of his phantasies and his terror of them was patent in many of his communications. Mostly the rays interfered with voluntary movement rather than with initiating aggressive outbursts or actions. This suggested that the rays also had a defensive role in so far as they limited the expression of the destructiveness which he felt within him. The conflict was well expressed in a statement that there were two kinds of thinking — Christian thinking and savage thinking. The former was peaceful and kind, whereas savage thinking was whatever used his eyes and body. Three or four sessions later he was mildly critical of the interviewer: but only for a few minutes. He returned to silence, only complaining that he felt as if he was being punched in the stomach. This symptom could be interpreted as resulting from a reversal of aim. Anger against the interviewer became self-directed.

The second test series occurred over five successive days. After the first test he told the interviewer that the rays now emanated from a machine — this was a new phantasy. He described this apparatus as a 'seeing machine'. It enabled the persecutors to see the same things as he was seeing. He added, 'They are able to reverse it so as to make things uncomfortable.' This was certainly a reference to the test apparatus, as the two lights did not switch on alternately; the right light was flashed successively before the appearance of the left light, and vice versa. Similarly, the auditory stimuli did not appear in a regular order. He did not attend for his next interview (the day of the second test session). He said that he had sprained his ankle and asked the interviewer to come to his room. He was more expansive about the machine and the rays: 'It can't continue like this because they are death-dealing weapons – they can kill you just like that.' Attempts to get him to elaborate on his experiences were of no avail.

The next day he said a little more about the machine – a second machine had appeared in front of him. This was causing a misdirection of the blood flow in his body. The machine appeared as a bright dome of light. He saw two discs in front of him which obscured his vision.

The psychologist reported that the patient refused to complete the test on the third day and did not attend on the fourth. He was, however, able to finish the test of the fifth and last day. He made the excuse that the rays interfered with his concentration and movement. On the last test day he told the interviewer that the persecutors had a new and terrible machine. They attached listening posts to his scalp – 'domes' which they fastened to his scalp to hold the veins. The 'domes' listened to the blood and made him feel weak. He felt very afraid.

In the interviews following the test he elaborated even further on his experiences. He explained, ' . . . They have rays which flash on to two points which are the main holding-points for movement (he indicated these points on the top of his head). They control the movement with thought from these two points. From the points veins go into the thalamus. The rays are mostly electrical but occasionally vibratory. The thoughts control the movement. They have spare parts. They have listening cones over the top of the head. They have fine rays and can be heard saying "right you've got it." There are three veins that go right down into the brain.'

After this he refused to continue the sessions because he could not leave his room. He attributed this to the rays. He was being attacked fiercely by a 'voice tube'. Attendants reported that since the testing his condition had become much worse. He was to be found immobile, complaining of intense bodily interference by the ray machines.

This patient's reactions demonstrated the powerful capacity of a test apparatus to provide both the stimulus for and the content of delusions. This man was frightened by his contact with the interviewer and it took a very short time before the delusional ideas entered the interview situation, thus rendering it of little value for the observation of the patient's subjective experiences. It was, however, within his capacity to deal with this anxiety.

Testing added an extra stress, which led to his refusal to continue coming to interviews. The test apparatus was endowed with a sinister significance. The phenomena indicate that the apparatus accentuated the fear of his omnipotent destructiveness. This threat could only be countered by muscular immobility. In these circumstances it would have been surprising if he had been able to continue through the testing without distress. It was indeed remarkable that he made so few mistakes on the three days he completed the tests.

Assimilation of the Experiment into the Delusional Complex

These four examples do not exhaust the list of psychomotor reactions to a test situation. There are other responses which must be mentioned, although detailed data will not in every instance be described. The first reaction worthy of mention is that provided by psychotic patients who exhibit delusions of grandeur and omnipotence. In Chapter 5 a reference was made to the fact that the content of delusions is not necessarily rigid and fixed although their core appears to be immutable. It was noted there that delusions can be responsive to new stimuli with a resultant assimilation of the new experience. This category of phenomena can be observed when certain patients are exposed to a test situation. In two cases that will be commented upon here, the effect of the test situation was to lead to the production of new delusional content.

The first is the man whose case (9) is described in detail in Chapter 5. After the second testing session he announced that the test apparatus itself had special qualities – that it was a special kind of scientific instrument designed to destroy the brilliant criminals. By an unknown technique these criminals extracted the essence of a man, leaving him an empty shell. This essence, whose physical manifestation was a double ('slips' or 'familiar' in another version of the delusion), could be transmitted from individual to individual. This patient's account of the 'slips', the double which every individual possesses and without which he is deficient in willpower, character, appearance, and ability to perceive the world meaningfully and with pleasure, is reminiscent of the ancient Egyptian concept of the Ka.

When the patient was seen after the second test he told the interviewer that the 'puppeters' (the criminals) were out of action. Everyone saw the surroundings in a different way and looked altogether better. He said, 'They're all free . . . they have got a different appearance . . . do you see the paint on the wall? Very much superior to what it was like when I was here yesterday . . . this wall looks as if it has been newly painted since then . . . you look much more human today.' *Interviewer:* 'How did I look yesterday?' *Patient:* 'Puppeting . . . you've still got the puppeting look . . . they all look much more human today . . . that Willie Smith (a patient) he looks much more human today . . .'

At a later interview he explained the cause of this change as follows. ' . . . All sorcery is dead again. Look out here (he stood up and walked to the window) — the doctor with his little machine put them dead . . . every time I put a light on (he meant pressing the key on the apparatus) it put them dead . . . (he then pointed out that the windows were cleaner and the paintwork was better) . . . even that corrugated iron . . . at times you almost wondered what it was . . . nebulous-looking you lose the waviness . . . that machine in there every time the red light that I am looking at to my right went on it killed them off because their opposition . . . not to me, not to the doctor but to the machine.' *Interviewer:* 'They were against the machine?' *Patient:* 'Yes . . . if you knew how to do it you could do all kinds of things with it . . . a machine like that . . . you have no conception the toy you are playing with . . . he works at it . . . but it's far more than he knows . . . it's far more than he knows himself . . . far more than the criminal thinks . . . he's doing something all the time . . . deliberately, purposively, wilfully, powerfully . . .'

A further case in which the experimental situation provoked the elaboration of delusional content was that of a male patient of twenty-nine who had been in hospital for about eight years. He entertained grandiose delusions which were often difficult to clarify because of defects in the form of his speech. Prolonged contact with this patient revealed that there were periods when his speech was almost normal and when the details of his delusional content could be noted (Freeman, 1962). The man believed that he had restored the hospital after it had been destroyed. He claimed a pension from the hospital on this account. He imagined himself to be a great poet.

When this patient was tested he condensed the test apparatus with a fire alarm outside the room in which the experiment was being conducted. This enabled him to regard the testing session as an extension of his activities in the hospital which he regarded as generally beneficial and helpful to all. This reaction could be interpreted as the means the patient adopted to avoid his anxiety about the apparatus and its purpose. A similar explanation might be employed in the previous case described. In favour of such an interpretation is the resemblance which such reactions bear to certain dreams of healthy individuals. In these dreams the dreamer is successfully engaged upon a dangerous task or the affective tone of the dream is cheerful and optimistic. Analysis of such dreams often reveals a latent content characterized by anxiety or depression. If this explanation could be substantiated it would add further weight to the theory that delusions have not only an adaptive function, as was described in Chapter 5, but a defensive function also.

It may be that when the defensive function of the delusion is maximally efficient the patient may be able to attend successfully to a task. However, the attentive capacity can be interfered with if the patient's preoccupations are so intense as to relegate the testing to a secondary role. This was so in Case 13 described in Chapter 6. Though this woman showed no clinical evidence of cognitive disorganization, she performed badly on the test. She told the interviewer that she was unable to concentrate because she was hearing a voice in her head. She also revealed that she expected to meet the hallucinatory object (a former man friend) in the room where the test was being conducted. To complicate matters further there are patients suffering from hallucinations — for example, Case 15 in this chapter — who can concentrate sufficiently well to perform a test adequately.

Many patients who were seen immediately after testing made no spontaneous comment about it. Even when they were asked about their reactions, they remained silent or had very little to say. In one or two cases it became apparent that they were afraid of the consequences of the test. One patient thought that the test was to find out whether she was fit for discharge — a prospect which frightened her very much. This absence of reaction on the part of patients suggests that such phantasies as had been activated are either suppressed or repressed.

The Experiment as a Vehicle for Displaced Anger

A final reaction that must be described is provided by patients who become angry and discontented with the interviewer or with the medical and nursing staff in general. This anger spreads to the test situation, leading to poor results. The following is an extract from the comments of an angry patient who had felt let down by the interviewer. He spoke as follows: '... you're wasting an awful lot of electricity — it's daylight and these lights on ... they wouldn't stand for it in C— mental hospital ... they wouldn't stand for it at all ... they've got lights on in that other room too ... I wonder if that girl is waiting to go in there ... (a patient waiting outside the interview room) ... she's probably a married woman ... did you get my Eldorado? (cheap wine) ... no money? ... surely you could spend half-a-crown at least ... surely a man of your standing could afford half a bottle of Eldorado wine ... the governor of a place like this cannot afford a bottle of whisky or a bottle of stout (sarcastically expressed).' Later he put his hands over his ears. When asked why he was doing this, he said, 'I've got a sore ear ... my ear has been burst, that f— doctor bursted it ... that gadget there in the other room, that noise, kept pressing the handles ten minutes or more in there.'

The reactions that have been described show that patients who are submitted to experimental procedures do not only respond in a general manner. Reactions are specific for each case. The external stimulus provokes phantasies of different kinds, which in some patients make their appearance in the delusions and hallucinations. It follows from this that the arousal of these phantasies can have a profound effect upon the patient's performance in the experimental setting. All the examples described indicate that the patient's reactions need not be confined to the test apparatus. The experimenter himself may become the stimulus and focus for phantasies of different kinds.

DISCUSSION

Attention must be drawn to the fact that the phantasies which arise in response to the tests are themselves conditioned by the predominant interests, conflicts, and preoccupations which are active within the patient. In one patient (no. 17) the test apparatus was used for the purpose of expressing phantasies that could not find an appropriate outlet. In this instance the reactions were derived from what amounted to a therapeutic relationship. It was a form of 'acting-out in the transference'. While these phenomena could be regarded as artificially induced — the patient having been seen regularly for a while before testing and thus developing strong transference reactions — it is important to recognize that patients who have had only minimal contact with psychiatrists may unconsciously carry transferences from their own family relationships into the test situation with results not unlike that described in Case 17. It is essential, therefore, that the investigator who employs special techniques in his research with mentally ill patients should be constantly aware that the test situation is a potent stimulus for psychic reactions with all the implications that this has for mental and physical performance.

The psycho-analytic forecast that a patient's behaviour in an experimental situation is not necessarily a response to the psychological or physiological stress has been confirmed in a number of recent reports. Several workers have demonstrated that the patients — not necessarily psychiatric — regard the unaccustomed situation of the experimental technique as a special stress. Sabshin, Hamburg *et al.* (1957) have shown that during the period of getting used to the laboratory setting anxiety and plasma hydrocortisone were raised and urinary hydroxycorticoids were as high during a pre-experimental day as they were later during experimental stress.

Lack of familiarity with respect to the experimental situation is therefore a stress in itself to which the patient reacts. This response may easily be confused with whatever reaction arises from the experimental stimulus. Schizophrenic patients are even more sensitive to experimental procedures. In support of this is Pollin's (1962) description of a study of psychological, physiological, and biochemical phenomena occurring during the infusion of adrenaline in schizophrenic subjects when compared with the reaction of normal controls (Pollin & Goldin, 1962). The schizophrenic patients differed from the control group in showing significantly more anxiety in response to the experimental situation but less in response to the adrenaline. The schizophrenic patients were much less able to cope with the experimental situation. As Pollin (1962) points out, without a comparison of the impact of the experimental situation upon the control and experimental groups, interpretation of the data obtained during the adrenaline infusion would have been misleading.

A somewhat similar observation has been reported by Tizard and Margerison (1963). Here, the frequency of generalized paroxysmal wave-spike discharges recorded from the two epileptic patients depended upon the content of the test situation. In a test which aroused the patients' interest or when watching the television, the frequency of such wave-spike discharges was much less than when the content of the test was dull and boring. The possible implications of this, when viewed from a psycho-analytic standpoint, are considerable because the state of boredom is one in which there is a proliferation of pre-conscious and unconscious phantasies. These reports (Pollin, 1962; Tizard & Margerison, 1963) indicate that it is not enough to consider whether a test result reflects the presence of a pathological mental condition. It is equally necessary to take into account the possible effects of the test or experimental situation on the performance of both physical and mental functions as reflected in physiological and psychological measurements.

It would appear, therefore, that, as psycho-analysts contend, not only do patients react — either physiologically or psychologically — to the content of an experiment, but they are equally sensitive to the general situation, which must inevitably include the person of the investigator. The psycho-analytic contribution to methodology lies in its assertion that the experimental subject will bring special mental reactions — in the nature of unconscious phantasies — into the experimental set-up and that these mental contents may have a decisive effect upon his response. It would be erroneous to envisage an experimental subject as an individual merely reacting to an unaccustomed situation. He will interpret the actuality of the investigation, first, in terms of his conscious preconceptions regarding research and, second, in terms of his unconscious phantasy life. This was quite apparent in the cases described in this chapter. The impact of the psychic reality may account in part for the psychological and physiological responses which appear during the course of experimentation.

CHAPTER 8

An Approach to the Classification and Diagnosis of the Functional Psychoses

It could be said that the purpose of the foregoing chapters has been to provide the foundation for what is now to follow — namely, an attempt to utilize psycho-analytic concepts for the diagnosis and classification of psychotic states. Psycho-analytic concepts may be divided into two overlapping categories. There are those which describe phenomena and there are those which are intended to delineate mental mechanisms that underlie specific mental functions or personality traits. The concept of resistance, which names a variety of phenomena encountered in the psycho-analysis of the neuroses, is an instance of the first category. Topographic regression is an example of the second, in so far as it does not describe a phenomenon (dream hallucination) but attempts to describe the mental mechanism that gives rise to it. It is concepts of the second kind that are most characteristic of psycho-analysis, because psycho-analysis is essentially concerned with trying to understand the psychological processes that underlie human experience and behaviour, whether normal or abnormal.

The psycho-analytic theory of psychosis employs concepts of the second variety. The concepts of cathectic disturbance, regression, and subsequent restitutional measures do not describe pathological phenomena but are an attempt to explain why they occur. The psycho-analytic approach to the psychoses is inevitably different from that of descriptive psychiatry in so far as the former is not committed to a model derived from organic medicine. The diagnosis and classification of organic disease are based upon an understanding of aetiology. Once this knowledge was gained it was possible to differentiate illnesses which had apparently identical symptoms. The causes of psychotic illness are unknown, and thus there are no means of clearly distinguishing one syndrome from another by means of special tests or investigations. The clinical psychiatrist has to classify a psychotic state and make a diagnosis solely on the basis of observable phenomena. His difficulties are accentuated even further by the fact that the phenomena mostly consist of the patient's subjective experiences and this increases the extent of observer error.

At the present time psychiatrists find it convenient to employ the classification of psychosis introduced by Kraepelin and later modified by Bleuler with his concept of the schizophrenias. This is no less true for psycho-analysis. Glover (1932) freely admitted his need to borrow concepts from psychiatric terminology when he constructed his psychoanalytic classification of mental disorders. Neither psychiatrists nor psycho-analysts are content with the descriptive method of classification and they are forever in a conflict between expediency and convenience and the desire to find a more satisfying and explanatory conception of psychotic illness. They find themselves forever having to accentuate one aspect of the phenomena and undervalue another in order to make the clinical phenomena fit the diagnosis. No one is satisfied with this state of affairs, but as yet there seems no better alternative. The psycho-analyst is not confined to this form of clinical categorization because of the essentially developmental nature of psycho-analysis. This has already been made explicit in earlier pages of this book.

It follows from the psycho-analytic theory of psychosis that, whenever a severe disorganization affects adult mental activity, phenomena of various kinds make their appearance as a consequence of the liberation of mental processes which ordinarily appear only in early childhood or in the dream. Even in the dream, their presence can only be inferred from the manifest content. Interspersed with the phenomena resulting from the disorganization are remnants of normal mental functioning. In addition, ideational content which has been acquired throughout life will be exploited by the emerging non-adaptive mental processes of the infantile period.

The psycho-analytic position could, if taken to an extreme, be put at the opposite pole from that of descriptive psychiatry. It could be said that whereas the former recognizes the variability of the clinical manifestations in psychotic states – manifestations which will be changing within the one patient and from patient to patient – the latter is committed to a number of fixed diagnostic groupings into which the clinical states must be pressed whether they fully accord with it or not. Such a comparison between the psycho-analytic approach and that of descriptive psychiatry does justice to neither. The nosological categories of descriptive psychiatry delineate clinical syndromes which enable the psychiatrist to classify psychotic states, but these groupings are, in practice, regarded as loose and approximate and not as definite entities comparable to physical diseases, where the area of involvement is accurately defined. The psycho-analytic approach has its disadvantages and dangers in so far as the phenomena which the illnesses present may be afforded less than their due importance. Emphasis can too easily be laid on theories without adequate regard for the phenomena upon which they should be based.

Psycho-analytic concepts of psychotic illness and the nosological scheme of descriptive psychiatry should complement one another. The latter approaches the clinical manifestations from the phenomenological standpoint and the former lays stress on the unconscious forces underlying the changing nature and content of the symptomatology. At the present time there is need for further attempts to find a better method of classifying psychotic reactions. This attempt is particularly necessary with the advent of chemotherapy in psychiatry. Today all psychiatrists know that the phenothiazine drugs can be of great assistance in the treatment of the individual psychotic patient. Unfortunately, every patient does not respond to these drugs, and the results of large-scale studies are often obscure and ambiguous. There are no agreed criteria for the administration of these medications, and no definite factors upon which the outcome of treatment might be forecast.

It is possible that information about these problems could be derived from detailed studies of individual cases. It is here that psycho-analysis may have an important part to play in helping to produce a better method of classifying psychotic reactions. One attempt in this direction has already been made by Ostow (1962), who has described a method of classifying patients in terms of libido economics. He has suggested that the phenothiazine drugs decrease the amount of libidinal energy available to the ego, whereas the monoamine oxidase inhibitors and iminodibenzyl derivatives increase it. He has described criteria of what he terms 'genital libido plethora' which characterizes certain psychotic states. Similarly, he has detailed characteristics of libido depletion. These concepts of ego plethora and depletion cut across descriptive categories and provide a basis for appropriate therapy.

A means of reducing the empiricism of drug therapy is by developing a more refined and comprehensive classification of psychotic states. Such a classification is theoretically possible by employing criteria that would identify clinical syndromes in a definitive way, thus establishing or refuting the identity of clinical syndromes currently diagnosed as nuclear schizophrenia, autism, schizo-affective states, atypical manic-depressive reactions, and mixed states. Similarly, the classification criteria should uphold or abolish the concept of the paranoid psychoses and that of the atypical depressive state.

In earlier chapters of this book, considerable attention was devoted to such concepts as object-relationship capacity, cognitive dysfunction, delusions, and hallucinations as they appear in schizophrenic states and paranoid psychoses. The purpose of this was to illustrate the manner in which psycho-analysis understands these phenomena, and thus to offer a number of criteria that may be used for classification. This attempt, like many others (Frosch, 1960) has much in common with the nosology created by descriptive psychiatry. This is inevitable because both approaches are attempting a definition of identical clinical manifestations, although using different conceptualizations. In this classificatory system, little emphasis is placed on whether the patient's illness could be diagnosed as manic-depressive psychosis, as paranoid psychosis, or as an atypical state. These nosological categories can be retained and employed alongside the analytic formulation. The classification criteria comprise: (1) object-relationship capacity, (2) affective reactions, (3) cognitive dysfunctions, (4) superego factor, (5) factor of defence, (6) hallucinations, and (7) delusions.

I. OBJECT-RELATIONSHIP CAPACITY

This concept was discussed at length in both Chapter 3 and Chapter 5. The position taken there was that all patients who suffer from psychotic illness do not necessarily retain the capacity for object relationships. This conclusion is based upon clinical observation and theoretical considerations. A distinction was made between a patient's capacity to react in a specific manner to the person of the psychiatrist or nurse and the presence of diffuse, non-specific responses which appear in all cases.

The appearance of discrete reaction patterns within the patient/ physician relationship is indicative of operating object cathexes. What is the nature of the cathexes which underlie these organized reaction patterns? This can only be inferred from the type of clinical data which is to be observed in the clinical situation. The first phenomenological

L

grouping is provided by patients who quite quickly manifest specific reactions to the person of the physician. Typical of this category of phenomena is the middle-aged patient (Case 5) discussed in Chapter 3 or the case of a woman of thirty who complained of auditory hallucinations and ideas of influence. Within three weeks of continuous clinical contact this patient had sexualized the relationship, coming to regard the interviewer as yet another who would use her for his own ends and then abandon her. This group of psychotic patients – often diagnosed as paranoid psychoses or atypical schizophrenias – frequently idealize the physician and attribute an omnipotence to him. These clinical data suggest that in these patients the organized reaction patterns are based upon residual object-libidinal (neutralized) cathexes and object cathexes of narcissistic type. Here the narcissistic organization is secondary in type and the cathexes are neutralized.

There is a second group of patients (see Chapter 5) who develop reaction patterns to the physician, but only through the medium of their delusional or hallucinatory objects. In these cases the physician and delusional object are condensed, thus indicating the activity of the primary process. It can be inferred that these reaction patterns are 'energized' by cathexes which belong to the primary narcissistic organization. These narcissistic relationships are to be distinguished from the (secondary) narcissistic transferences described for the first group. The 'primary' narcissistic cathexes are instinctual in quality, freely mobile, and operate under the laws of the primary process.

Finally, there is a third group of patients who do not react in an organized manner (Cases 7 and 10, Chapter 5) and in whom an absence of any form of object cathexis can be inferred. They react in a non-specific manner in an interpersonal situation, and it is suggested (Chapter 3) that this is due to the appearance of a level of mental functioning in which object, needs, and self are inextricably fused. In such cases the cathexes are disorganized and wholly turned inwards upon the fragmentary self-representations. These are the patients variously described as autistic (see Chapter 10), or as cases of dementia praecox or nuclear schizophrenia and in whom there are severe disorders of speech form, neurological disorganization, and disintegration of the self and the sense of identity.

In Chapter 3 attention was drawn to the observation that when psychotic patients enter a regular treatment relationship two separate series of phenomena appear related to the interviewer himself. First, there is the displacement of psychotic phenomena into the interview situation. These reactions may consist of misidentification of the therapist, confusion of patient with the interviewer, negativism, and persecutory delusions. These displacement phenomena can be compared with the 'floating' transferences which are to be noted at the outset of psychoanalytical treatment and were referred to in Chapter 3. Psychotic phenomena, on the one hand, and floating transferences, on the other, are not peculiar to a treatment situation and can as easily be displaced to friends, employers, or in the case of patients to nurses or doctors. Second is the development of special forms of specific reaction to the therapist. In some cases these patterns are based upon object-libidinal cathexes, as described above.

There are, then, a number of identifiable patterns that may arise in the course of a clinical contact with a psychotic patient. The organized responses are to be distinguished from the generalized non-specific, diffuse reactivity that may appear in every case whenever the patient is brought into contact with a clinician, nurse, or occupational therapist. It is implicit in this conceptualization of the clinical phenomena that the detection of an object-relationship capacity cannot be undertaken in the course of one or two interviews. The patient requires to be seen daily for at least three or four weeks, and detailed information must be obtained from nurses and attendants, who also offer themselves as objects onto whom cathexes will be directed if they are available to the patient.

This formulation, although based on psycho-analytic concepts, is implicit in the diagnosis and classification of descriptive psychiatry. The clinical psychiatrist is aware of the importance of the patient's ability to relate and the extent to which the volitional function is retained. Unfortunately, this knowledge is not always made explicit nor is it sufficiently recognized that it takes time for information about this function to become available

2. AFFECTIVITY

The second factor that must be assessed is the state of the patient's affects, often a difficult problem in psychotic states because of withdrawal and lack of interest. Affective phenomena in psychosis can be classified with less doubt and ambiguity if they are understood as derivatives of the instinctual drives. The physiological and psychological manifestations that constitute affects can be regarded in the healthy as reflecting the status of the drives. This does not apply to patients suffering from psychoses. The cases that present an apparent lack of affect may be those in whom the drive towards objects is largely in abeyance owing to the disorganization and de-neutralization of object cathexes.

Affective reactions are not a reliable index of the presence of the object-relationship capacity. The view has been put forward that object-relationship capacity (transference potential) is synonymous with an advanced level of mental functioning to be distinguished from a general tendency to react to the stimulation of interpersonal contact. In Chapter 2 an account was given of the psycho-analytic theory of affects (Rapaport, 1953) which emphasizes that an increasing control is exerted over the affects as development proceeds. Fine regulation of affect and object-relationship capacity go hand in hand in the healthy adult. In abnormal states the organized capacity for object relations has been lost and all that is left is a diffuse reactivity. In such cases the affects, like the reactivity, are uncontrolled and unmodulated, appearing to act as if their function was governed by an 'all-or-none' law.

When the affective reactions of psychotic patients are examined in terms of this theory, it becomes clear that they cannot be regarded as primary factors for either diagnosis or classification. It follows that the form and intensity of affective expression will first and foremost be a consequence of the extent of the mental disorganization. In cases where the mental disorganization is minimal, affective manifestations will not show the liability or intensity that will occur where the disorganization is extensive. It is in the latter group of cases that a sudden swing can occur from an absence of affect to an affective explosion. In such instances it would appear as if the affects, having lost their regulatory mechanisms, are held in abeyance by poorly organized – often motor (muscular) – controls and that minimal stimuli lead to affective discharge.

Hyperactivity in the physical sphere is usually accompanied by the expression of affects of all kinds. Unregulated affectivity can occur in association with any form of psychotic phenomenon. At the other end of the scale – where affect seems to be lost – motor activity is limited and there is a diminution of interest in the environment. These manifestations are also non-specific and can occur with different constellations of psychotic symptoms.

Affective reactions are an intrinsic part of every mental illness, hence the diagnosis and classification of a psychotic reaction must depend on the presence or absence of factors other than the affects. One of these factors has been described (object-relationship capacity) and others will be detailed below. It is well known that serious mental disorders may initially present with affective disturbance and it is only later that other manifestations make their appearance. In such cases an insight is provided into the role played by the affects, but of great significance is the fact that the affects are not the decisive process that leads to the psychotic condition. The affective reactions are secondary to the disruption of the patient's object-relationship capacities. The following is a case in point.

CASE 19. The patient was a single woman of twenty-eight who was admitted to hospital suspected of suffering from a schizophrenic state. While nursing her father she had become withdrawn, depressed in mood, and self-preoccupied. On one occasion she threw tea at a little niece of whom she was extraordinarily fond. At another time she jumped out of bed and wanted to dance with her father, but within seconds accused him of wickedness and sexual misdemeanours. It came to light later that she had discovered that her father was having a sexual relationship with his housekeeper. At this time there was no observable evidence of delusions, hallucinations, or cognitive dysfunction.

Within a few weeks the patient's condition settled and she was discharged from hospital. However, she was admitted a few weeks later in a state of excitement. She told the doctor in charge of her case that she was in love with him. She wanted to be with him all the time and she showed all the signs of a sexual interest. For the next eighteen months a therapeutic relationship was maintained with this doctor. During some of this time she was out of hospital. Her mental state fluctuated between periods of well-being and periods when she was extremely depressed, self-reproachful, and self-critical. At this time a diagnosis was made of manic-depressive psychosis. On one occasion she attempted suicide and had to be brought to hospital in a semiconscious state. Most of her self-criticisms related to sexual phantasies, none of which were revealed at the time but which were probably due to transference. In addition to expressing these self-reproaches, she was constantly worried about her appearance.

Unfortunately, the doctor who was treating the patient left hospital. It is conceivable that the events now to be described may have been causally related to the separation. Gradually the patient began to express the fear that she had venereal disease. Then followed the statement that she had had a miscarriage in hospital and was receiving poison-pen letters saying she was lewd and lascivious.

One afternoon while watching a cricket match in the hospital grounds she suddenly realized that one of the cricketers was responsible for the poison-pen letters. She now saw herself as the subject of an organized persecution. This primary delusional idea was followed by a host of accusations against the doctor who had looked after her prior to his leaving the hospital. She said that he had assaulted her sexually and injected her with venereal disease. Within a few months similar accusations were levelled against the medical superintendent. She complained that it was his intention to turn her into a prostitute. She said that her hatred of the medical superintendent was due to the fact that he looked like her father.

She continued with these accusations over a period of many months and during this time expressed the belief that, as a child, she had witnessed her father having intercourse with her mother. She accused her father of brutally beating her and subjecting her to unnatural practices. The recollection of parental intercourse was paralleled by the accusation that the medical superintendent was having a sexual relationship with the matron. During all this time she was difficult to manage because of a negativistic and aggressive attitude.

As the months passed she became progressively more grandiose, the culmination came with the announcement that she was Princess Victoria Louise, a daughter of George VI. She told the ward sister that when she was young she had been sent to live with the man and woman she had believed to be her father and mother. From this moment on she refused to communicate with any of her family, and her attitude towards other patients, doctors, and nurses was arrogant in the extreme. She broke into violent rages when addressed by her real name and constantly asserted that doctors were twisting her brain and doing everything within their power to prevent her from having her true identity revealed.

For a long time she was unapproachable, and it was only when she was induced to undertake treatment with chlorpromazine that the delusional ideas completely disappeared. From this time on she became accessible to influence but still retained a number of symptoms, among which were headaches, difficulty in relating to others, upset of vision, and a general loss of emotion. It is of interest that following the initial injection of chlorpromazine she told the nurse that the drug had damaged her genitalia and made her morally loose. Later, when she was no longer preoccupied with the delusional ideas, she insisted upon a psychological examination because of her fear that the drug treatment might have damaged her intellectual functions.

This patient's illness began when she discovered that her father was having sexual relations with his housekeeper. It is likely that the proximity of this sexual activity stimulated latent masturbatory phantasies. The initial reactions were twofold. First, the ego organization was affected in the area of its defensive functioning against the drives. For a brief period the patient acted erotically towards her father. Second, superego anxiety ensued, expressing itself in a condemnation of her father, a preoccupation with religious ideas, and a depression of mood. The ego defect rapidly disappeared and the patient appeared to have recovered. The recovery was assisted by the attachment she had developed for the doctor.

At the next admission the ego defect had reappeared. Repression had failed and the sexual drives had the doctor as their object. Once again the ego recovered its defensive functioning and her reactions were for some time predominantly superego in type. The suicidal attempt indicated the extent of the patient's aggression, although at this time it was dealt with by introjection into the superego.

Continuous contact with the doctor who had seen her at the first admission provoked intense transference phantasies. Guilt and anxiety resulted from the hate provoked by disappointment. This accentuated the severity of the superego, leading to the suicidal attempt. It may be hypothesized that when the doctor left the hospital the patient reacted with intense disappointment and rage. Introjection of these impulses into the superego created a degree of guilt feeling that the patient was unable to master without reverting to a far-reaching regression. This regression was also facilitated by a fresh failure of the ego defence directed against libidinal drives. Such a hypothesis found support in the fact that it was after the doctor left the hospital that the patient announced that she was pregnant and complained that the latter had infected her with venereal disease and meningitis.

Her later behaviour indicated that she gradually withdrew interest from the world of objects and concentrated her attention upon the new delusional ideas (restitution). A regression to a pathological narcissistic state had occurred. This regression would account for the multitude of sexual and other bodily sensations that plagued the patient. It was on the day of the cricket match that projection of her guilty wishes and phantasies took place for the first time. From then on, projection and denial (see Factor of Defence, p. 165) had the functions of defence. The construction of the delusion helped the patient to come to terms with the alteration in her bodily sensibility created by the narcissistic regression.

Only at a later stage did the psychotic narcissism declare itself openly in the grandiose delusions whose content belonged to the category of the family romance. At this stage the narcissism was absolute. It was as if the whole of the libidinal cathexis was involved in the self and none was available for objects. Throughout this patient's illness oedipal conflicts were uppermost. They precipiated the illness, they continued their existence in the transference relationship, they were lived out in delusions of persecution, and finally they appeared in the form of a delusional family romance (Freud, 1909).

In this case the affective reactions were the outward manifestation of an underlying disturbance that did not reveal itself until an intolerable stress was placed upon the patient's capacity to relate. When her object cathexes became disorganized, an attempt was made to reconstruct a new reality on the basis of childhood daydreams, but their sadistic quality led to anxiety and guilt with resultant distressing experiences. This case shows how a patient's clinical state must be examined and categorized at different phases of the illness. Here, affective manifestations were paramount in the first episode of illness but later they were of secondary significance to the fundamental derangement of the object-relationship capacity.

3. COGNITIVE DYSFUNCTIONS

All psychotic states are characterized by a disturbance of cognition in the spheres of judgement and insight. The presence of this defect is indeed the principal criterion for the diagnosis of a psychotic reaction. Apart from this, cognitive dysfunction may be entirely absent, as with the majority of depressive states, or present to an obvious extent, as in patients usually diagnosed as suffering from hebephrenic schizophrenia.

The investigation of a patient's cognitive status consists essentially of determining how far the different mental processes that make up the ego organization diverge from the level at which they would operate were they engaged in a task necessary for environmental adjustment. Such tasks demand the employment of attention, concentration, perceptual processes, judgement, and intact memory schemata. The patient's capacity for sustained attention and concentration is assessed during the clinical interview by estimating the ease or diffi-culty with which extraneous and internal stimulation is inhibited.

The examiner must be constantly on the lookout for the occasional intrusion into the stream of talk of fragments of overheard phrases and apparently random visual percepts (see Chapter 4). It is not only the intrusion of extraneous percepts which is of importance, but also the patient's capacity to isolate the contents of his thoughts from the sub-ject-matter taken up during the course of the psychiatric interview. There are patients who report that they are unable to describe the details of, for example, a picture, because of the constant pressure of associations from within. Such a patient finds that images, words, and ideas lead involuntarily to floods of thoughts which prevent him from continuing with the directed aim of his thinking.

The capacity to attend is closely linked with perceptual processes, and here the examiner must be concerned with estimating the patient's capacity for discrimination. In the visual field evidence must be sought indicating, first, a loss of the ability to discriminate one individual from another; second, the condensation of current figures with those from the patient's present or past life; third, the ability to discriminate perceptual modalities. Patients have been observed in the acute phase of an illness who could not discriminate between auditory and visual percepts (Chapman, Freeman & McGhie, 1959). Then there are other cases in which figure and ground are fused and visual perceptual constancies are lost.

In the sphere of bodily awareness, observation must be directed to-wards finding out whether the patient can at all times discriminate himself as an entity from other individuals. One woman patient believed that she was growing a moustache like her husband, and she similarly confused the doctor with him. Another female patient had the idea that her sister's body had entered her own body, leading to a change in the shape of her hips. As in a dream, the patient represented her fear of becoming as lascivious as her sister by believing that she was becoming like her physically.

Disturbances of bodily awareness and spatial orientation are fre-quently encountered in psychotic states. The phenomena include defective localization and discrimination of body parts; complaints of changes in weight, size, and shape of limbs, head, and trunk; perception of the body outside the self (Schilder, 1950; Bychowski, 1943). Denial (extinction) of tactile and kinaesthetic sensations and faulty discrimina-tion of tactile and postural stimuli are also to be found. In some instances the stimuli are located outside the body. A number of authors have suggested that a similarity exists between these phenomena and the abnormalities of the body scheme (Critchley, 1953) that characterize lesions of the parietal lobe (Angyal, 1936). It is also of some interest that disorganized psychotic patients and patients suffering from parietal lobe lesions (Critchley, 1951) show a similar form of inconsistency in their response to the one examination technique.

The investigator is dependent upon the verbal utterances of the patient for knowledge of the functional state of the thought processes. He is therefore at a disadvantage, because he can never really pass beyond inferences about the nature of the thought processes themselves. Nevertheless, the change in form which the verbal representations take is sufficient to enable him to identify phenomena indicating the presence of a thinking disturbance. Such phenomena as the inability to sustain a train of thought, or unintelligible or illogical associations, are not in themselves pathognomonic of any one mental illness, but may be encountered in a number of different conditions. A difficulty arises from the absence of criteria that can be taken as reliable indices of a formal disturbance of thought. As far as possible, speech defects should be described separately from abnormalities of thinking.

During the clinical interview, the examiner must inquire whether there is evidence of a disorganization of concept formation. This disorganization finds expression in the aberrant or primitive forms of concept, examples of which have been given in earlier chapters. Attention must equally be given to phenomena indicative of a breakdown in the representational function — where objects and abstract ideas are no longer represented by the appropriate verbal symbols. This failure is apparent in the familiar situation where thinking is less dependent upon the meaning of a word than upon its sound and concrete pictorial significance. Failure of the representational function is also to be found in the fragmentation of verbal ideas, which leads, among other consequences, to the *pars pro toto* phenomenon. Associated with it is the concretization of words and parts of words. This results in patients talking and using a word as if it were an important possession or plaything (see Chapter 5).

All these manifestations must be regarded as the result of a process affecting cognitive functioning in such a way as to lead to de-differentiation, primitivization, and disorganization. The outcome is the appearance of a general tendency towards the condensation (Freud) or syncretism (Werner) of mental processes that were previously discrete and autonomous. The discriminatory defects that have been described are not usually of a crude and obvious nature, as they are in patients who are confused to time and place, but appear only sporadically in the course of the patient's communications.

An account of cognitive disorganization would be incomplete if reference was not made to yet another important result of dysfunction in this area. There are patients who complain that people are talking about them and behaving strangely towards them. They can often give details of what is said. In such cases there is no evidence of hallucinatory phenomena, and the observer is forced to the conclusion that these patients are selecting and misinterpreting their perceptual experiences. It would appear that the discriminatory mechanisms which ensure a veridical perception of the environment are in abeyance. Cases of this kind are usually diagnosed as paranoid reactions or paranoid psychoses to distinguish them from schizophrenic states.

This clinical differentiation is justified on a number of counts. First, these irrational beliefs can be understood as resulting from the intensification of a process which occurs, in special circumstances, in the mentally healthy. It is a common experience in conditions unfavourable to accurate perception for individuals to come to erroneous conclusions about environmental events. The clinical phenomena described represent a perversion of the mechanism of 'inductive belief' referred to in Chapter 4. Second, these misinterpretations are limited in extent and are not associated with irrational ideas related to special methods of persecution, interference with bodily functions, or with auditory hallucinations. It is, of course, true that cases which eventually show all the signs of a nuclear schizophrenia may begin with misinterpretation and only gradually do the more serious phenomena make themselves manifest. Further discussion of these paranoid psychoses will be undertaken under the heading 'Delusions'.

The presence of widespread cognitive disorganization is of decisive importance for the categorization of a psychotic state. Cognitive disorganization can be associated with a partial capacity for object relations. On the other hand, cognitive dysfunctions can occur with a complete detachment and withdrawal from the environment. This series of clinical phenomena (cognitive dysfunction) does not necessarily indicate a bad prognosis. It is well known that patients exhibiting many such manifestations rapidly recover. Reference has already been made to the observation that it is cases of this kind which support the classical theory that cognitive disorders are secondary phenomena. The presence in mental hospitals of chronic psychotic states in whom the cognitive dysfunction remains static over many years suggests that there may be, in addition, a group of cases in which the cognitive disorder is itself a primary defect.

4. SUPEREGO FACTOR

A classification of the functional psychoses based on psycho-analytic theory is impossible without invoking the concept of the superego. The self-reproaches and self-criticisms of depressed patients are regarded as resulting from the pressure of a 'hypertrophied' superego. In the majority of depressive illnesses it is the principal dynamic factor and one into which the patient has no insight. His judgement is defective in this respect. There are, however, a number of patients in whom self-criticism exists alongside the belief that they are being criticized by those about them. This criticism may or may not be considered justified by the patient. Here is an illustration of the manner whereby the interpretation of the perceptual world is influenced by conative factors. The patient attributes (projection) superego attitudes to those about him. He then selects and misinterprets what they say and do in order to fit in with his own beliefs about himself.

Cases in which there is a projection of the superego are more seriously disturbed than those in which the criticisms are recognized as arising within the self. It is less common today to find delusional ideas, hallucinations, and cognitive dysfunctions associated with self-reproach, but this can occur, as in the following case of a woman of forty-six. She expressed elaborate and irrational self-criticisms into which she had no insight. She believed that she had plunged the world into war. She showed evidence of thought disorder in so far as she was unable to pursue a theme to its conclusion. She was hallucinated, expressing grandiose delusions to the effect that she received messages saying she was God. Interestingly enough, this patient remained depressed in mood throughout the illness and was never elated or over-active. She misinterpreted events in favour of her self-condemnation – people disliked and criticized her. All this was due to the fact that she had brought humanity to disaster.

Before proceeding to a description of other clinical states in which a projection of the superego occurs, it is worth recalling that the superego has at its core elements of what Freud originally called the ego-ideal. Freud (1914) went to some lengths to demonstrate that the ego-ideal — the physical, ethical, and intellectual aspirations of an individual — has its origins in the narcissism of childhood. He contrasted sublimation — the displacement of the aims of the instinctual drives from direct bodily satisfactions to intellectual or moral satisfactions — with the aims of the ego-ideal, which normally bear little relationship to an individual's real capacities. He demonstrated that the aims of the ego-ideal are based on wishful phantasies and on an omnipotence of thought. Too great a discrepancy between real capacities and ego-ideal aspirations can lead to feelings of hopelessness and depression of mood.

Recognition of the omnipotent wishes that lie at the core of the superego helps to explain certain aspects of patient symptomatology which arise from an externalization of the superego. Two categories of patient can be recognized in this respect. First, there are those who believe that others are criticizing them and this is based upon mis-interpretation alone. Then there is the second group, who are convinced that others have the power to read their thoughts or arrange the en-vironment in such a way as to test out their integrity. Though such patients are self-critical, the attribution of magical powers to those about them indicates the activity of a projected superego which has regained its infantile narcissism (omnipotence). Finally, there are those patients in whom the superego is not only projected but also fragmented. In such cases the patients complain that they are criticized and persecuted by numerous individuals and the criticism is normally by hallucinatory voices.

Projection of the superego in any of the forms described above can occur in any psychotic syndrome. It may be associated with con-siderable cognitive disorganization or cognition may be wholly intact. Similarly, it may be associated with depression of mood or with an apparent absence of effect. Again, the patient may be utterly with-drawn from the environment or still be able to make meaningful relationships. It is unnecessary to discuss in detail those patients whose clinical state alters from being criticized (projection of superego) to self-criticism and vice-versa. A second group who show changes in the function of the superego are those in whom self-criticism alternates with criticism and aggression against others.

5. FACTOR OF DEFENCE

Patients suffering from psychotic states can also be classified in terms of the defence mechanisms employed in the course of the illness.

The defence mechanisms described by psycho-analytic theory are not regarded either as identical in their function or as on a similar organizational level. It is generally assumed that repression is the most stable and highly organized of the defences. Repression is a mechanism that operates efficiently and effectively only after the infantile period has passed, by which time the ego has achieved some degree of coherence and stability. Other defence mechanisms equivalent to repression in organizational complexity are reaction formation and secondary identification. The latter process is the means whereby personality develops through the introjection of attitudes, ethical standards, ideals, and the behaviour of admired persons. Secondary identification is a selective mechanism, in contrast to primary identification, which belongs to the earliest infantile period and describes the indiscriminate assimilation of environmental experience.

Displacement, denial, projection, introjection, reversal of instinctual aim (active to passive), and regression (topographic) are mechanisms that lack the stability of repression, secondary identification, and reaction formation. They are brought into play when necessary and then allowed to lapse. This is easily observed in the healthy, where projection or displacement may be transiently employed under the stress of anxiety or guilt. Repression, though also available for such emergency measures, has essentially an enduring quality, thus allowing the exclusion of the potentially disruptive and disturbing conative tendencies of earlier periods of life. It is important to remember that in the neuroses repression is not completely damaged in its function. According to psycho-analytic theory, there is a partial failure of repression and it is this which leads to a break-through of the repressed. This distinction between the neuroses and the psychoses is important when assessing the nature of the defences in the psychoses.

In Chapter 2 an account was given of the theory that in the psychoses the cathexes which underlie object-relationship capacities change in their nature. The object cathexes become replaced by narcissistic (instinctual; deneutralized) cathexes. This means that the self becomes of significance at the expense of objects. It is also hypothesized that the regression to a narcissistic form of mental organization is facilitated by the fact that the infant passes through a phase of primary narcissism in which there are no separate objects and no cathexes to innervate them. This is the period of primary identification.

It follows from this aspect of the theory of psychosis that a return to a narcissistic organization will lead to the activity of mental mechanisms appropriate to that organization. Such mechanisms are reversal of instinctual aim, 'turning in on the self', and topographic regression. Increased concern with the self will create a predisposition for drives to turn back on the self whenever they meet with the obstacle provided by anxiety or mental pain.

Psychotic reactions can be classified in terms of the extent to which repression remains operative. This can be gauged by the presence or absence of direct instinctual actions which ordinarily remain unconscious or confined to the realm of thought. An example is provided by Case 19, when the patient impulsively and out of character threw a cup of tea at her little niece. A further index of seriously defective repression is the appearance of displacements and condensations (primary process) affecting the cognitive functions thus leading to a disorder of thought (faulty concept formation) and to misidentifications, self-object fusion in the perceptual sphere. Inappropriate affective responses and outbursts of uncontrolled affect also suggest the presence of totally inadequate repression.

In patients who show extensive or limited defects of repression other defences also operate. Cases characterized as paranoid psychoses, depressive psychoses, and mixed states are generally those in whom repression and reaction formation remain relatively intact. It may be that here projection is employed to avoid further stress upon the repression barrier, and thus repressed phantasies and the superego are exteriorized. This leads to the misinterpretation of perceptual experiences described under Cognitive Dysfunction (p. 163). Projection is one of the most commonly employed mechanisms in psychotic states that are free of serious cognitive disorganization. Introjection of both object and drive is another frequently encountered mechanism in conditions in which there is little personality deterioration. Such a mechanism predominates in the depressive psychoses.

The distinction made in Chapter 5 between psychoses characterized by well-formed delusional complexes (paranoid psychosis, paranoid schizophrenia) and those in which there is a generalized disorganization of all mental functions (dementia praecox) is supported further by the following observations. There are patients in whom repression, far from being ineffective, appears to be in the service of the trend towards the organization of a new reality. These patients insist that they have no awareness of their current situation, even denying knowledge of the name of the hospital or that they are in a hospital at all. In certain cases they complain of having forgotten their real names, and inquiries reveal that everything associated with the illness, its onset, and course, has been entirely repressed. A more agreeable explanation of the patient's position is substituted for the memory lapse. These repressions are accompanied by denial, and the phenomena bear the closest resemblances to those denials of bodily incapacity which sometimes accompany organic cerebral disease (anosognosia) (Weinstein & Kahn, 1950). The employment of repression in the manner described only occurs in patients in whom the ego organization is still functioning in a fairly effective manner.

Reversal of instinctual aim, turning in on the self, and topographic regression are seen most clearly in cases where repression has lost its function of defence and where the ego organization is in a state of disintegration. Cases 7, 8, and 10 described in Chapter 5 are good examples of this development. These mechanisms also operate in cases where repression is still functioning but there it is less apparent, being overshadowed by the activity of repression, projection, and introjection. It is the delineation of the predominant defences which gives a clue to the principal unconscious conflicts. Although delusions will be discussed in detail below, it is worth recalling that the defence mechanisms do not create delusions, but merely determine their content. Projection, denial, and reversal play an important part in this respect, as has been seen in the cases described.

In those cases generally categorized as paranoid schizophrenia, projection has a special character, which must be designated psychotic in order to distinguish it from the projection that occurs in the mentally healthy and in the psychoneurotic individual. In psychoses patients employ projections to disown responsibility for actions, wishes, affects, thoughts, and images. The question is whether the two forms of projection are to be distinguished on a purely quantitative basis or whether they are qualitatively distinct. A strong case has been made for the view — particularly by psycho-analysts — that psychotic projection with its compulsive quality is wholly a product of regression. Does this explanation apply to every instance of psychotic projection? There are reasons for thinking that this is not so.

The content of psychotic projections is often made the basis for a clinical distinction between paranoid states (paranoid psychosis) and paranoid schizophrenia (see below — 'Delusions'). It is those patients who complain of induced motor and sensory changes who are most likely to be diagnosed as suffering from paranoid schizophrenia, in contrast to those who say that they are forced to think or feel in certain specified ways. In the former category, emphasis is placed on alterations of bodily experience, whereas in the latter complaints are confined to the mental sphere. The sensory experiences include changes in the position of the body *vis-à-vis* external space, rotatory movements, faulty location of tactile stimuli, defective postural sense, and unusual sensations of weight or lightness. An accompaniment of these experiences is an awareness of another alien individual from whom the patient cannot clearly differentiate himself. This leads the patient to report that the actions he performs are not done by him.

It is conceivable, as was suggested by Schilder (1928) and more recently by Chapman and McGhie (1962), that in those patients who are so profoundly disturbed the psychotic projection and its content are both an integral aspect and a secondary reaction to alterations in cerebral function. A number of investigators have pointed to the fact that many of the sensory experiences reported by psychotic patients are similar in many respects to the results of lesions affecting the parietal and temporal regions of the brain. Such an explanation does not entirely invalidate the regressive hypothesis as long as it is understood that the defective brain function has found expression in childhood. It may be, as is so often the case, that psychotic projections and their appropriate contents should not be regarded as either wholly organic or wholly psychological in origin. An explanation that includes both factors must offer the most satisfactory means of classification. A scale can be envisaged, at one end of which the psychological factor predominates, with organic involvement minimal or absent. At the opposite end, the organic factor is paramount. Between the two poles, various combinations of the two factors will be found.

6. HALLUCINATIONS

Hallucinations were discussed in detail in Chapter 6, where they were divided into two categories depending upon their relationship to objects. One category comprised those hallucinations which had the function of creating a new reality and were therefore restitutional in aim. In such instances the hallucinations had been split off from objects to which they were originally related and thereafter continued in an autonomous state. The content of these hallucinations depends upon the patient's cognitive status. In those who show disorganized thinking, the hallucinatory content may consist of neologisms or words which are used inappropriately.

M

The second category of hallucinations comprises those which remain tied to the object. The various functions these hallucinations may undertake were discussed in Chapter 6. The fact that hallucinations, whatever their ultimate function, originally arise as the consequence of disturbances in the sphere of object relations is the basis upon which the psycho-analytic theory of hallucination is founded. According to this theory, hallucinations derive their cathexes from accumulated instinctual energy which has failed to find an outlet in motor activity. Hallucinations are drive-cathected ideas — memory traces brought to a hallucinatory quality by the activity of the drives. They are treated by the patient as identical with the drives and their derivative phantasies. If the drives provoke anxiety and guilt, then the same reactions follow the appearance of the hallucinatory experiences. In this respect hallucinations constitute a form of the return of the repressed. This instinctual aspect of hallucinations has been pointed out by Katan (1950), who regards their function as principally one of instinctual discharge.

7. DELUSIONS

Reference has been made above to the misinterpretations which psychotic patients make of their perceptual experience. The misinterpretation was ascribed to defective perceptual discrimination resulting from the presence of repressed conflicts. These irrational ideas usually have a persecutory content. In the group of patients concerned, the irrational beliefs never extend beyond an exaggeration of what is possible in fact — namely, rumours are being circulated which blacken the patient's reputation. There is little of archaic or infantile phantasy in these preoccupations. An example is that of a fifty-two-year-old single woman who, after a hysterectomy, believed that the surgeon had told people that she suffered from venereal disease. The idea was later elaborated to the length of her being an immoral person. At no time did she believe that her mind was being influenced or controlled and she was never hallucinated.

These patients must be distinguished from those in whom the delusional content consists of phantasies which can only be described as archaic or infantile in nature. The phantasies may be wishful or persecutory. Not only are individuals or powers of some kind working against the patient but the persecutors employ all kinds of secret, magical, or scientific means to interfere with his mind and body.

Clinical psychiatry makes a distinction between the two categories on a purely descriptive basis, describing the former as paranoid psychoses and the latter as paranoid schizophrenia. Psycho-analysis adds a further means of distinguishing them. According to this theory, the first category of irrational ideas is not principally concerned with restoring relationships with an environment from which the patient has been torn. He retains this contact, and the clinical manifestations represent an attempt to reconcile instinctual demands with the limitations imposed by anxiety, guilt, and the restriction set by reality.

In the first category a regression of the instinctual organization has occurred in order to bring about a solution of a conflict, and this leads to the appearance of a pathological narcissism — that is, to a state of exaggerated egocentrism where the omnipotence of thought is restored. Ideas have a greater reality than the reality of the environment. Cognition remains intact in a structural sense, but it is influenced by the narcissistic regression thus leading to misinterpretations. The patient remains in this new position *vis-à-vis* his relationship with the environment. There is no attempt to develop a new reality nor do the irrational ideas serve as a means of external adjustment. Close examination of these patients generally reveals that the symptoms arise from conflicts regarding specific individuals to whom the patient is inextricably bound. These individuals eventually turn out to be the 'reincarnation' of the objects of childhood. Paranoid states, depressive psychosis, and mixed states are the nosological labels usually attached to cases of this type.

Within the first category there is another group of patients, often similarly diagnosed, in whom attachment to the world of objects appears to be more precarious. Here the delusional content consists primarily of a dread of the effect of imagined destructive powers. This may extend from those near to the patient, to physicians, to nurses and it may sometimes include the world itself. These patients do not create a new reality through their delusions and hallucinations — rather they misinterpret environmental events to satisfy their need (often unconscious) for punishment on account of their feared destructiveness.

Though having certain phenomenological characteristics in common with the first group of patients, the second category of cases shows additional and unique features, some of which have already been mentioned. Differences are also to be found when the phenomena are examined in terms of psycho-analytic theory. The delusions have, as their main function, the aim of creating a new reality. They give meaning to the mental and physical experiences which the disease has induced and they act as a method of adaptation.

At the outset of the illness it is possible to discern interpersonal conflicts that relate to the delusions, but with the passage of time these ideas are elaborated on and come to substitute for the abandoned reality. The patient described at the beginning of this chapter illustrates this kind of development. The appearance of a primary delusional idea was associated in time with an upset in an interpersonal relationship. Thus far there was a similarity between this patient's state and that of patients belonging to the first category. However, further developments led to the appearance of new psychical constellations comprising childhood (family romance) phantasies, erotic preoccupations stemming from the oedipal period, and attitudes arising from the disintegration and projection of the superego. The delusional complex became the patient's object world.

Delusional ideas, like hallucinations, can, therefore, be divided into those which are predominantly restitutional in function and those which are attempts to solve conflicts that have arisen in relationships to which the patient is still tied. In the latter group the construction of the symptomatology is along the lines of the psychoneurotic symptom, in so far as the phenomena represent the outcome of a defensive conflict. The delusional idea, like the hallucination, may be a means of countering the pain of object loss or of neutralizing anxiety and guilt arising from the activation of forbidden drives. In the restitutional group, the delusions are not related primarily to conflict – they are the end-product of an object-relationship conflict that has been given up. It follows that the two categories described here represent extremes of a range, and therefore many intermediate varieties will occur. Only the detailed study of cases can lead to the data being accurately located along this range.

According to the scheme just outlined, all patients suffering from functional psychoses can be classified along seven dimensions – namely, object-relationship capacity (transference potential); affective reaction; cognitive status; superego factor; factor of defence; nature of hallucinations; and delusional data. This form of classification cannot be adequately undertaken unless the patient is studied closely over a number of weeks. By this method it is possible to estimate at what point on each dimension the phenomena are to be located. If it was thought desirable the information could be recorded in a quantitative manner by the construction of appropriate scales.

It may be thought that this form of classification is static in nature and does not take into account the unconscious conflicts which relate to the phenomena. While there is some justification in such a criticism, it is preferable to remain close to phenomena currently observable rather than to have recourse to inferences regarding conflicts that may have existed prior to the onset of the illness. To some extent the deficiency implied in this criticism is offset by the importance attached to the recording of data relating to the object-relationship capacity and to defence. Conflicts and defences tend to reappear in relationships with clinicians and nurses and there an opportunity is afforded of observing and recording such data.

Patients can be classified at different phases of the illness or before and after the employment of special medications. This classification, based upon descriptive and psycho-analytic concepts, takes full account of the variations that characterize psychotic phenomena. It helps to overcome the inevitable tendency to trim phenomena to fit in with nosological entities. It acknowledges the originally tentative nature of the original diagnostic groupings. There is no reason why conflict should exist between this approach to classification and that traditionally employed by clinical psychiatrists. Both can be used, although that described here may have a greater value for research in prognosis and therapy.

Before the dimensions forming the classificatory scheme can be employed, it is necessary to specify criteria that characterize their upper and lower limits. Object-relationship capacity (transference potential) can be scored as present only when definite evidence is obtained of a specific pattern of object-relationship behaviour, as has been described in earlier parts of this book. Allocation of the patient on the affective dimension will depend upon the extent to which the affects are controlled and still retain their capacity to function as signals. Lack of affective control and disorganization *vis-à-vis* ideation will give a low position on this dimension. As far as cognition is concerned, allocation on the scale will depend upon the extent of the cognitive disorganization. A patient's place on both the superego and the defence dimensions will be dependent upon the organizational level at which the functions represented by these concepts operate. Projection and fragmentation of the superego will place the patient low on the scale, as will the predominance of defences of low organizational stability. Hallucinations and delusions will be sited in accordance with their functions, as has already been described.

On the basis of this scheme, a patient suffering from dementia praecox whose symptoms could be envisaged as completely static (a purely hypothetical construct) would rate low on all the dimensions, whereas a patient diagnosed as a manic-depressive psychosis would rate high on nearly all the dimensions. Such hypothesized states do not, of course, correspond with the realities of clinical experience. The employment of dimensions acknowledges the changes which may take place in the functional level of mental processes in psychotic illness. It also indicates that the classification of a psychotic state cannot be made on the basis of only one or two positive clinical findings.

It is a regrettable fact that this is what frequently happens in research projects designed to study aspects of the schizophrenia problem. Very often the group of patients which are designated schizophrenic is a heterogeneous collection of clinical states in which delusional complexes are the only common feature. The evidence advanced to substantiate the presence of auditory hallucinations is usually weak in the extreme, and they are not clearly differentiated from misinterpretation of overheard speech. Little attention is given to the state of the object-relationship capacity beyond some reference to volitional disturbance, catatonic phenomena, impulsiveness, or negativism – all non-specific phenomena from a diagnostic standpoint. No distinction is made between those patients who retain, in some degree, the object-relationship capacity (paranoid psychoses, atypical manic-depressive states) and those in whom it is reduced to non-specific reactivity. Details of affectivity and cognitive dysfunctions are frequently neglected.

The identification of a schizophrenic psychosis requires not only the unequivocal presence of serious damage to the object-relationship capacity but also the appearance of delusional complexes and hallucinations that are serving restitutional aims. Whatever it is that underlies these phenomena leaves the patient remote, detached, and without regard for either himself or those around him. Concern for others is enough to contra-indicate the diagnosis of schizophrenia. This is essentially the position of leading British psychiatrists (Hill, 1962; Batchelor, 1964) who are unwilling to designate a psychotic state as schizophrenia as long as the patient retains interest and affectivity. All delusions and hallucinations do not have a restitutional function and thus cannot be regarded alone as indicative of a schizophrenic illness. This diagnosis should only be made whenever all the factors listed are affected in the manner detailed earlier in this chapter. Failure to take them into account usually leads investigators to advance unwarranted conclusions regarding the aetiology, the pathophysiology, the psychopathology, and the clinical course of schizophrenic psychoses.

The essential feature of the classification presented in this chapter is the attempt to accommodate diverse phenomena that make their appearance during the course of a psychotic illness. It is this phenomenological variation which bedevils descriptive psychiatry. Psychiatrists are constantly being confronted with patients who present phenomena that should be absent if they are to fit into a particular syndrome or who exhibit signs without the other data with which they should be associated. A classification based on psycho-analysis deals more easily with the observable data and the changes to which they are subject.

CHAPTER 9

Psychological Studies of Schizophrenia

A chapter dealing with psychological studies, which are predominantly experimental, may appear at first sight rather out of place in a book with a frankly psycho-analytical approach. During the last decade, in the United Kingdom, a marked schism has developed between the two disciplines of psycho-analysis and clinical psychology. This has been due in part to the experimental nature of much contemporary psychological research in the clinical field, which had led many psychologists to eschew psychodynamic formulations as being outside the limits of their declared brief of objectivity. While psychologists criticized the unwillingness of the psycho-analyst to examine the validity of his operational concepts, the psycho-analyst in turn scornfully rejected the experimental approach as being naïve and sterile. The divergence of the two disciplines was ironic in its timing, coming as it did at a period when psycho-analysts such as Hartmann (1951) and Schachtel (1954) were widening the original tenets of psycho-analytic theory in a direction that could more easily accommodate the findings of psychological research. Recently, however, there have been indications that authorities in both fields are becoming more willing to consider past criticisms of the limitations of their respective approaches. '. . . There is some evidence that psycho-analysts tend to abstain from applying such reliable controls as are available, with the result that views gain currency and sanction on hearsay evidence. The *ipse dixit* acquires the validity of an attested conclusion, largely by a process of repetition . . . There is in fact little discrimination in the psycho-analytic field between controlled research and individual opinion, which cannot always be distinguished from unchecked speculation.' This, and other equally frank and critical remarks, were made recently, not by any of the avowed opponents of psycho-analysis, but by Edward Glover (1964), a leading British exponent of psycho-analytic theory. While the psycho-analyst has admitted the need to subject some of the basic psychodynamic formulations to controlled and systematic scrutiny, some experimentalists have expressed dissatisfaction with the often superficial nature of an approach that achieves a spurious sense of objectivity only by severely limiting its field of inquiry. In a recent dissertation on the development of experimental psychology, Professor Oliver Zangwill of Cambridge (1964) declared, 'It soon becomes apparent that human reactions are influenced by internal no less than by external circumstances, and that experimental control of the former is difficult, if not impossible, to achieve. Thus although the stimulus applied to an individual may be controlled with the utmost precision, we cannot so readily control or determine the mental attitude which he brings to its interpretation'. Such views are very much in accord with the suggestion made by Dr Freeman in the introduction to this book that the two approaches of contemporary psychology and psychoanalysis are complementary in so far as each may act as a corrective to the particular limitations inherent in the other.

Dr Freeman's assertion is particularly relevant to the experimental studies in which the present writer has been involved, in that these investigations had their roots in psycho-analytical observations. Some years ago I had the pleasure of working with Dr Freeman and Dr Cameron in a clinical study of groups of chronic schizophrenic patients. Although this investigation was psycho-analytic in its conceptual and operational framework, the intensive study of chronic schizophrenic patients led us to reject the idea that schizophrenic symptomatology could be regarded as being due primarily to unconscious conflict over interpersonal difficulties. We concluded (Freeman *et al.*, 1958) that the basic disruption in the psychic life of these patients was in the area of ego functions. A further comparison of the chronic schizophrenic patient's behaviour with that of the young child (Freeman & McGhie, 1957) gave support to the view that these very deteriorated patients operated at a perceptual level comparable to the primitive and unorganized state characteristic of infancy and early childhood.

The task of differentiating between the different forms of ego disturbance observable in chronic and very deteriorated schizophrenic patients is, however, fraught with difficulty. The relative inability of these patients to communicate directly and to describe their subjective experiences in a comprehensive manner necessitates an attempt by the observer to unravel the, superficially meaningless, manifest content of the patient's verbal and non-verbal behaviour. The validity of such interpretations of psychotic behaviour depends greatly on the observer's therapeutic skill and knowledge of the individual patient, and the dangers of subjective contamination and error may go unchecked. Apart from the inaccessibility of the chronic schizophrenic patient to direct examination, we are faced with the difficulty of distinguishing between behaviour that reflects the end-state of a psychotic disease process and that which is a result of chronicity due to prolonged hospitalization. A detailed study of a single case of a schizophrenic patient (Chapman *et al.*, 1959) illustrated to us how the young schizophrenic patient at an early stage of his illness is able to describe more directly the subjective changes which he is currently experiencing. In a later clinical study of twenty-six early cases of schizophrenia (duration of illness ranging from six to eighteen months), a standard interview was used to encourage the patients to describe, in their own words, recent changes in their experiences. In presenting the clinical data collected in this way (McGhie & Chapman, 1961), the authors attempted to arrange the patient's reports under categories which, as nearly as possible, reflected the main areas of cognitive disturbance suggested by the reports themselves. The disorders of ego function, most frequently mentioned by these patients, included a variety of perceptual changes, defects in the comprehension and production of speech, an inability to control and direct the course of thinking, and changes affecting movement and motor responses in general. There was, however, one other category of change experienced which not only outweighed all others in the frequency with which it was reported, but was also described as the earliest change subjectively noted by the patients themselves. This we referred to as a disturbance in the selective and inhibitory functions of attention, which caused the patients to be pathologically distractable. The patients expressed this disability in different ways, but the following extract from one patient's description is fairly typical of their statements. 'I can't concentrate. It's diversion of attention that troubles me ... The sounds are coming through to me but I feel my mind cannot cope with everything. It's difficult to concentrate on any one sound ... It's like trying to do two or three different things at the one time.' To deal effectively with the environment, the ego function of selection must operate so that, out of the mass of information relayed via the sense organs, only that which is relevant to the task at hand enters consciousness. This process of selection applies also to the diverse series of images, memories, and associations that make up our internal environment. Our patients' reports suggested that they were no longer able to make such selective responses and that their perception, thinking, and actions were being continually disrupted by this inability to inhibit or screen out sensory data unconnected with their current activity.

In reviewing the contribution of psycho-analytic studies of schizophrenia, Dr Freeman (1958) suggested that it may soon be possible 'to undertake a systematic mapping out of the state of ego functions in patients suffering from schizophrenia.' Thus far our clinical approach had allowed us to go some way in this direction, but many questions remained unanswered. For example, are these disorders of attention, perception, memory, motility, and other ego functions uniformly present in all schizophrenic patients? Do such disorders occur to some degree in other psychiatric conditions, or in normal subjects? To what extent is the quality and degree of such disorders related to the severity or duration of the schizophrenic illness? In order to answer these and many other questions raised by the clinical observations, it was necessary to provide a more objective way of assessing the degree to which the disorders of selective attention were present in the patients studied. The most satisfactory method of approaching such a task was to utilize the controlled methodology of the experimental approach. This does not imply that experimental findings are by their nature automatically more valid and more reliable than clinical observations. Clinical observations may provide their own internal criterion of validity *if* they are made in a controlled and systematic way. Perhaps the main justification for translating clinically derived observations to an experimental setting is that we thereby provide some safeguards against over-enthusiastic speculation. Finally, it might be as well to remind ourselves at this point that it is the initial clinical observations on patients which generate the hypotheses capable of being experimentally assessed. The experimental method allows us to extend these hypotheses and examine specific variables in greater detail than is possible in a purely clinical setting.

Most of the remainder of this chapter will be used to describe and discuss the experimental investigations we have carried out in recent years, and some of the clinical inferences we have drawn from our findings. These studies are essentially concerned with the effect of distraction on selected areas of schizophrenic performance, their main aim being to allow a more careful delineation of the disorders of selective attention reported so frequently by schizophrenic patients. To date, these studies have embraced a total of sixty schizophrenic patients, forty controls with a non-schizophrenic psychotic illness, and sixty normal subjects. We are also currently examining the performance of patients with a clearly definable organic disorder, but the results of this comparative study are not yet available. Our earlier analysis of the subjective reports of schizophrenic patients suggested to us that the following spheres of ego functioning were most frequently affected by the schizophrenic disease process: (i) perception and immediate memory; (ii) psychomotor performance; and (iii) language behaviour. It may therefore be more convenient, and I trust more coherent, if we initially consider the studies under these three categories. We shall then attempt to draw together the results of these and related studies reported by other workers in the form of a rough model of the type of ego dysfunction which these investigations suggest to be characteristic of schizophrenia. Finally, we shall consider the more difficult question of whether such experimentally derived results provide any useful information in helping us to deal with the individual schizophrenic patient within a therapeutic relationship.

THE EFFECTS OF DISTRACTION ON PERCEPTION AND
IMMEDIATE MEMORY

In our first attempt (Chapman & McGhie, 1962) to bring under experimental examination the deficit in selective attention reported by schizophrenic patients, we used a number of techniques designed to assess the influence of distracting stimuli on the patient's perceptual performance. One of the most successful of these techniques consisted of a simple visual tracking test, in which the subject was shown a ciné film of a white spot moving randomly to the right or left of a central position. The subject's task was to track the lateral movements of the spot by means of a hand-operated lever, his responses being automatically registered on an electric pen-recorder. Distraction in this test took the form of a high-pitched buzzing noise, introduced from time to time to the left or right ear through split earphones. From a comparison of the performance of schizophrenic patients with that of non-schizophrenic patient controls and with that of normal subjects, it was found that the introduction of the distracting stimulus had a very marked effect on the schizophrenic group. When asked to perform the test in the absence of the distracting stimulus, the schizophrenic patients greatly improved their performance. The striking deterioration in the performance of schizophrenic patients on this type of task suggested that distracting auditory stimuli may directly affect the act of perception. A number of the patients did, however, comment that the distracting stimulus had affected, not their perception of the moving spot, but their inability to hold the correct lateral movement of the spot in their mind long enough to allow them to make the appropriate response. These comments implied that the effects of distraction might be exerted chiefly in the brief period between perception and response, and that the main influence of distraction was on short-term memory.

To investigate this possibility further, we have carried out a number of studies in which the influence of distraction on immediate memory was examined more directly. The basic technique was to present the patient with a simple series of stimuli, usually rapidly presented letters or digits, together with a similar series of irrelevant pieces of information. The patient's task was simply to observe and report back the relevant series while ignoring the irrelevant information. In some of these tests the relevant and irrelevant information were both presented in the same sensory modality, whereas in the others two sensory modalities were involved. Thus the subject might be presented with sequences of digits or letters recorded by a female voice, and simply asked to report each sequence in the correct order immediately after completion. In some sequences the interval between each two items was filled by an irrelevant number or letter recorded by a male voice, which the subjects were instructed to ignore. The difference between the subject's basic score on this task without distraction, and his score on the sequences containing irrelevant material, was expressed as a proportion of the basic score. The resultant 'distraction index' thus represented the extent to which the subject's performance was affected either positively or negatively by distraction. A similar technique was used to assess the effect of visual distraction on visual performance, and finally, the subject was asked to carry out a comparative task where the distracting stimuli were presented in alternate sensory modalities. In this latter task, the subject would be presented with auditory and visual sequences simultaneously and instructed to report back only the sequences presented in one sensory modality. These tests were specifically designed to examine the subject's ability to screen out and ignore information which was defined as irrelevant, either by its physical characteristics or by the modality in which it was presented. Subjects were also tested in a somewhat different situation which demanded the integration of information derived from two sensory channels. Here, the subject was asked to perceive and briefly retain sequences of letters and numbers, the individual items of which were presented alternately in the auditory or visual channels. This auditory-visual integration test allowed us to compare the subject's recall score for the auditory and visual parts of each presented sequence separately.

Analysis of the data obtained from these and later experiments (McGhie *et al.*, 1965) indicated that, in the tasks in which the subject is asked to attend selectively to auditory information, performance of the schizophrenic patients is markedly affected by distraction, whether this distraction occurs in the auditory or the visual modality. In tests where the main task is that of selectively attending to visual information, it was found that the introduction of auditory distraction had again a marked effect specific to the schizophrenic group. The introduction of visual distraction in those tests involving visual attention had, however, no particular effect on any of the subjects, including the schizophrenic patients. It would thus appear that the ability of the schizophrenic patient to attend selectively to visual information is affected by auditory distraction, but not by distraction in the visual modality. The negative result of the test which assessed the effects of visual distraction on visual performance, is, however, possibly an artifact based on the nature of the tests used. The irrelevant distracting visual stimuli were spatially separated from the relevant information and peripheral rather than central attentive adjustments would tend to figure more prominently in this task. In examining our data further it was, however, noted that the schizophrenic patients tended to perform poorly on all tasks involving the perception and recall of visual as opposed to aural stimuli, irrespective of whether or not distraction was present. A good initial performance on the basic visual tasks without distraction would tend to mask the effects of distraction on the later parts of the test. Again, in the auditory-visual integration test where the patient is required to utilize information in two sensory modalities, the errors made by schizophrenic patients tended to be confined to the visual component of the test. In other words, when asked to perceive and recall a sequence comprising auditory and visual stimuli, schizophrenics have particular difficulty in responding to the visual elements in the sequences. We have found a similar modality difference to occur in another type of test used recently to study the interaction between the auditory and visual components of immediate memory (McGhie *et al.*, 1965a). Again, it was evident that schizophrenic patients have particular difficulty in the short-term retention of visual as opposed to aural information. The possible reasons for such modality differences will be discussed later in this section.

Thus far we have spoken of the schizophrenic patients as if they could be treated as a homogeneous group. Most studies of schizophrenic patients, whether clinical or experimental, reveal that this is hardly the case and that the generic term 'schizophrenia' embraces a highly heterogeneous sample of patients. This heterogeneity was clearly evident in the performance of our schizophrenic patients on the tests which we have used. Before being tested, each patient in our studies was given a standard interview to obtain data on his present clinical state, his previous history, and his premorbid personality. This interview material was later transferred to a rating scale to allow us to extract from the schizophrenic group those patients whose psychosis had taken a more severe and malignant form. The patients who were given high ratings on this clinical scale tended to show a markedly schizoid premorbid personality, to have had a long and insidious onset to their illness, and to have shown in their current symptomatology marked flattening of affect and thought disorder. The majority of the schizophrenic patients in this subgroup had been diagnosed as hebephrenic, and closely compared in their clinical state to Kraepelin's original picture of dementia praecox. For convenience of classification this group of 'nuclear' schizophrenics will be referred to simply as hebephrenics. When these patients were compared with the remainder of the schizophrenic group, it was clearly evident that it was the hebephrenic subgroup who tended to show the higher degree of distractability. It was also evident that the presence of systematized delusional thinking was negatively related to distractability as measured by our tests. A later comparison with a group of psychotic patients diagnosed as suffering from a paranoid psychosis, substantiated this suggestion in that these patients were found to be no more distractable than the subjects in the normal control group. Finally, the schizophrenic group was subdivided in terms of chronicity. Using the arbitrary cutting-off point of five years duration of illness as a standard of chronicity, we made an analysis of the scores based on this division which showed a slight tendency for the chronic patients to be more distractable; but the difference between the performance of the chronic and the remaining schizophrenic patients was by no means marked and in no case statistically significant.

These studies, then, appear to offer some support for the original clinical hypothesis that schizophrenic patients demonstrate a marked disorder of selective attention. This relative inability of the schizophrenic patients to screen out irrelevant extraneous information was seen to have a particular effect in situations which demand the accurate perception and recall of information. Further analysis of the test findings indicates that this disorder is not evenly distributed within the schizophrenic group, but tends to be concentrated among the patients whose psychosis has taken a more severe and malignant form and who may be categorized as hebephrenic.

THE EFFECTS OF DISTRACTION ON PSYCHOMOTOR PERFORMANCE

In the reports given by schizophrenic patients, many of the comments suggested that distraction, particularly in the auditory modality, tended to interfere with the smooth sequence of their motor responses. In order to investigate this suggestion in a more systematic way, we constructed a battery of eight tests each involving some aspect of psychomotor performance. These tests were all essentially speed tests involving speed of response in simple motor tasks (e.g. finger tapping) or in reaction to simple stimuli (e.g. simple reaction time). The tests were constructed in such a way as to allow the effects of both auditory and visual distraction on test performance to be examined independently. When the schizophrenic patients were compared to non-schizophrenic patients and normal controls, it was found (McGhie *et al.*, 1965b) that the basic psychomotor functioning of the schizophrenic patients was clearly inferior. This is, of course, not unexpected since the majority of these tests involved speed of motor response and it is now well established (Payne, 1961) that psychomotor retardation is a common consequence of psychotic illness. However, although auditory and visual distraction affected the performance of the psychotic patients as a whole, these experiments did not support the initial hypothesis that the disruption in performance was more pronounced in the case of schizophrenic patients. Further analysis did not reveal any differences in performance between the different clinical subtypes of schizophrenia, nor was there any evidence of distraction exerting a differential effect on chronic as opposed to acute schizophrenic patients. Most of the tests used in this investigation required simple motor responses to predictable stimuli. However, in a few of the tests, which were slightly more complex in that the subject had to respond quickly to a stimulus occurring at varying intervals (e.g. simple reaction time), there was a tendency for the schizophrenics to be somewhat more affected by distraction. The Spot Tracer test described earlier also involved a motor response to a variable and uncertain signal and here, it will be remembered, schizophrenic performance was extremely vulnerable to distraction. The tests used in our experimental inquiry required only repetitive and simple motor responses where speed of response was the deciding factor. It would be interesting to compare schizophrenic patients in their performance on more complex psycho-motor tests in which decision-making was involved.

THE COMPREHENSION OF SPEECH IN SCHIZOPHRENIA

On interviewing schizophrenic patients, we had previously observed that a number of them repeatedly declared difficulties in their compre-hension of speech. The following comment made by one young schizophrenic patient is typical of the behavioural change reported by many: 'When people talk to me now it's like a different kind of lan-guage. It's too much to hold at once. My head is overloaded and I can't understand what they say. It makes you forget what you've just heard because you can't get hearing it long enough. It's all in different bits that you have to put together again in your head — just words in the air unless you can figure it out from their faces.' Careful examination of such reports suggested that they resulted not from the patient's inability to perceive the individual words comprising a connected discourse, but from a deficiency in perceiving the words in meaningful relationship to each other as part of an organized pattern. This 'de-patterning' effect is perhaps more suggestive of the disorder found in dysphasic patients but we found it to be reported with a high degree of frequency by our schizophrenic patients. Until Shannon's (1948, 1951) investigations of the statistical structure of language, there was no satisfactory method available which would allow objective assessment of the factors involved in the 'depatterning' of speech. Shannon showed that, in normal English, letters are not used with equal frequency, and letter combinations are even more restricted in their occurrence. The extent to which the occurrence of any letter is governed by the letters which precede it, presents a measure of what has been called contextual constraint and may be expressed in terms of transition probabilities between letters. For example, given the letter A, the probability of its being followed by N is quite high, whereas the probability of its being followed by K is fairly low.

The statistical structure of words in context can be similarly described. Miller & Selfridge (1950) constructed a series of passages of English words exhibiting varying degrees of contextual constraint. The first passages in their series contain no contextual constraint, the words being unrelated and selected at random. The final passages are taken from standard English texts and therefore represent the highest degree of contextual constraint possible. The intervening passages are graded according to the degree of contextual constraint involved in their structure. The following two passages represent the second and seventh orders of contextual constraint for ten-word passages.

1. Was he went to the newspaper is in deep and.
2. Recognize her abilities in music after he scolded him before.

Presenting this series of passages to a small group of normal subjects, Miller & Selfridge showed that the ability to recall these passages immediately after presentation improved steadily as the order of approximation to ordinary English increased. In other words, the subjects showed themselves able to utilize the increasing degrees of contextual constraint (internal organization) of the passages to improve their performance.

It was decided to utilize this method in order to examine objectively the conclusions drawn from the clinical data on the speech difficulties of schizophrenic patients. For the purposes of this experiment, two testable hypotheses were advanced pertaining to the performance of schizophrenics on a task involving the recall of meaningful material:

1. Schizophrenic patients will be less able than normal subjects to improve their performance by utilizing increasing degrees of contextual organization.

2. Schizophrenic patients will perform nearly as well as normals in their recall of material with no contextual constraint (i.e. randomly selected words).

When passages were presented to schizophrenic patients, the results (Lawson *et al.*, 1964) confirmed that the patients were able to perceive and recall those sentences with a very low order of contextual constraint as well as did normal subjects. The schizophrenic patients, however, failed to improve with the succeeding passages of increasing contextual constraint. In other words, the patients appeared to be unable to utilize the transitional bonds between word units which allow the normal person to perceive the passage as an organized whole.

Investigations are at present under way to assess the effect of contextual constraint on different lengths of passages, and we are also using an equivalent test to assess the subject's ability to utilize increasing degrees of contextual constraint in the perception of visual stimuli.

It has been shown that passages involving contextual constraint contain redundancy, in that some of the words are almost entirely predictable from their context, so that the measure of contextual constraint represents a measure of redundancy. The ability of the normal subject to increase his recall score for the constrained passages can be interpreted as demonstrating his ability to screen out the redundant material and only retain those parts of the passage necessary for adequate comprehension. Such a process of redundancy reduction may well be analogous to the process whereby irrelevant stimuli from the environment are inhibited, so that the schizophrenic patient's difficulty in speech comprehension may reflect his failure to attend selectively. It is at least theoretically possible to apply this type of approach to schizophrenic speech production. Laffal (1961) has already applied such an analysis to the language of a schizophrenic patient, and Herdan (1958) has used a somewhat similar technique in analysing the vocabulary of dysphasic patients.

A MODEL OF DISTURBED ATTENTION IN SCHIZOPHRENIC STATES

The conclusion that schizophrenic patients demonstrate an inability to attend selectively to incoming information has been reached independently as a result of a number of other studies of schizophrenic performance. Weckowicz & Blewett (1959), in a series of investigations of changes in perceptual constancy in psychotic states, found evidence for reduced size constancy in schizophrenia and were later able to show that such perceptual anomalies were positively correlated with thought disorder. In seeking to interpret the clinical significance of their experimental feelings, Weckowicz & Blewett argued that perceptual constancy depends on the ability to process the perceptual cues in the environment in such a way as to exclude those cues which are irrelevant and would lead to inaccurate perception. In reviewing their findings, they concluded that, 'the abnormalities of thinking and perception in schizophrenic patients could be described as an inability to attend selectively or to select relevant information'. Venables and his colleagues (1959, 1962, 1963), in a series of studies of the arousal level of schizophrenic patients, also concluded that many of the behavioural ab-normalities shown by these patients were due to variations in the range of attention. Discussing his experimental findings in acute schizo-phrenic patients, Venables explained many of their difficulties as being related to 'a broadened level of attention which causes the patient to be overloaded by sensory impressions from the environment'. On the basis of many years of experimental investigations of schizophrenic performance, Shakow (1963) reached the following conclusions: 'It is as if, in the scanning process which takes place before the response to a stimulus is made, the schizophrenic is unable to select out the material relevant for optimal response. He apparently cannot free himself from the irrelevant among the numerous possibilities available for choice. In other words, that function which is of equal importance as the response *to* stimuli, namely, the protection *against* the response to stimuli, is abeyant . . . These irrelevant associations . . . would appear to arise from three sources: chance distractors from the environment; irrelevancies from the stimulus situation; and irrelevancies from past experience . . . The mere presence of these irrelevant factors seems to lead the schizophrenic to give them focal rather than ground signifi-cance, signal rather than noise import.' Payne and his colleagues (1959, 1960, 1961, 1963), in an extensive series of studies of psychotic thinking, have been able to show that the thinking of the schizophrenic patient may be differentiated from that demonstrated by other psychotic patients by the factor of 'overinclusion'. Overinclusive thinking is seen by Payne to represent, not a thinking disturbance at all, but as a more basic disorder affecting the attentive processes: 'The mechanism of attention itself seems to become defective. Whatever filtering mecha-nism ensures that only the stimuli (internal or external) that are relevant to the task enter consciousness and are processed, seems no longer able to exclude the irrelevant. This has numerous repercussions. Thinking becomes distracted by external events. It also becomes distracted by irrelevant personal thoughts and emotions which may even become mixed up with the problem. Selective perception becomes impossible, so that instead of dealing with the essence of the problem, irrelevant aspects are perceived and thought about . . . '

Studies of early ego development by psycho-analysts and genetic psychologists have already afforded us some insight into the develop-ment of this 'filtering mechanism' of selective attention. The original Freudian notion of an undifferentiated ego-id, close in conception to Piaget's state of primary adualism, indicates that the first stages of life are characterized by an undifferentiated protoplasmic consciousness in which there is no distinction between the self and the outside world. In this state, where inner mentality and outer reality are fused in one global whole, it would appear that the infant passively assimilates experiences in an undifferentiated fashion whether these experiences originate in the external environment or within his own body. In order to obtain subsequent control over his environment, the developing infant must learn, not only to discriminate between different environmental stimuli, but also to select and organize the incoming flow of sensory stimuli. Thus, to a large extent, the differentiated ego develops by a process of selection and inhibition of incoming sensory data, so that only part of the whole sensory background is effectively registered in consciousness. For this development to take place we must postulate an internal mechanism which allows the organism to select from the diffuse sensory input the information necessary for it to function effectively.

Recent advances in neurophysiological studies point to the role of the brain stem reticular activating system in carrying out this essential operation of selective monitoring of incoming information. In surveying the relationship of the reticular system to the process of attention, Brain (1958) declared: ' . . . it looks rather as though its (the reticular system) function were to prepare not only the cortex but the other sensory pathways also to respond to a sensory impulse when it has arrived. As we have seen, such responses are at least twofold, namely the reduction of other sensory "information" which might compete for attention, and the integration of the sensory "information" being attended to with the continuously changing background of somatic and environmental sensory data'.

A psychological model of attention incorporating the concept of a filter mechanism has been developed by Broadbent (1958) and used extensively by him in his experimental studies of human communication. Broadbent's model is that of a single decision channel with a limited capacity for handling information. In order to overcome the limitations inherent in this system, a filter operation is performed on its input. Broadbent and his colleagues have demonstrated that the probability of any data being selected to pass through the filter depends on certain attributes of the stimuli in question and upon the current state of the organism. This work has also made it clear that the limitation of the human communication channel is an informational one, so that the number of stimuli we can respond to at any time is determined by the amount of information they contain. It is thus possible to deal with more than one set of data at a time only if the informational demands of each task are small. In order to function effectively, the individual is forced to select and process information in such a way as to avoid overloading his limited capacity to deal with it. Broadbent's experiments have demonstrated that, where information is presented at a rate above the individual's maximum capacity for dealing with it, performance breaks down.

The experimental studies of schizophrenia indicate that the normal processes of selection and inhibition governing attention have broken down so that these patients suffer from a marked inability to attend selectively to stimuli in such a way that only relevant information is processed. In dealing with situations that require responding to simple, predictable stimuli, overloading is less likely and the patient's deficit less obvious. In tasks where the subject is required to monitor a range of stimuli involving more complex decisions which occupy the limited decision channel, the failure in selective attention leads to overloading and consequent breakdown in performance. The suggestion that the performance of schizophrenic patients is particularly poor when visually presented information is processed, may possibly be explained by recent findings (Sperling, 1960; Conrad, 1964) that visual data are usually recoded into the auditory modality before storage. This translation process appears to impose a further strain on short-term retention and creates a further source of error and confusion in schizophrenic performance. The 'depatterning' effect observed in the disordered speech perception of schizophrenic patients may be regarded as a further aspect of the general disorder in selective attention and short-term memory. The accurate perception of speech requires the processing of a much greater amount of information than that contained in the rather simple and artificial situation represented by most of our tests. Normally, we are able to handle this greater amount of information by organizing the data into larger speech units, thus reducing the load on short-term memory. In speech perception we are greatly aided by our automatic use of the transitional bonds which exist between words in normal language structure, so that the screening out of the redundant words which occur in most verbal communications is possible. The schizophrenic seems to be less efficient in his ability to organize the incoming verbal stimuli in an economical way and unable to direct attention away from the redundant words. Whether he is able to overcome these disabilities and deal effectively with verbal communications will depend on such factors as the rate at which the verbal data are presented and the amount of information which they contain. In the next and final section of this discussion we shall consider some of the practical consequences of this deficiency in dealing with verbal communication in a clinical setting.

While recent psychological studies are largely in accord in their conclusion that some schizophrenic patients show a primary deficit in attending selectively to incoming information, there is less agreement as to how this deficit is distributed within the heterogeneous group of patients who are given the diagnostic label of schizophrenia. Shakow (1963) and Weckowicz & Blewett (1959) concluded from their studies that schizophrenic patients with pronounced paranoid symptoms showed very little evidence of impaired selective attention, this impairment being confined to the hebephrenic group. Our own findings also suggest that it is the more disordered hebephrenic patient who demonstrates a marked impairment in selective attention. Other workers, however, notably Payne (1963) and Venables *et al.* (1962, 1963), have argued that a high degree of distractability is more characteristic of patients with marked paranoid symptoms – and is particularly noticeable in the acute phase of the illness. These contradictions are probably due less to genuine differences in the experimental findings than to the manner in which these findings have been interpreted. The clinical difficulties in establishing a reliable differential diagnosis of the various subtypes of schizophrenia must also be an important factor in accounting for these contradictory conclusions. It is fairly obvious that additional investigations, based on careful and reliable clinical assessments, are required to allow us to define more precisely the relationship between experimental findings and schizophrenic symptomatology.

THE APPLICATION OF EXPERIMENTAL FINDINGS TO
THE THERAPEUTIC HANDLING OF SCHIZOPHRENIC PATIENTS

As we have noted earlier, the experimental investigations we have outlined were originally derived from clinical observation of schizophrenic patients receiving psychotherapeutic treatment along psychodynamic lines. It would be extremely satisfying if we were able to transfer information derived from the experimental work back to its original clinical setting, particularly with regard to the psychotherapeutic handling of schizophrenic patients, and in this section we shall explore this possibility.

Our investigations so far have allowed us to go some way in drawing a rough map of the disorders of ego function in schizophrenia, although the outline is still very sketchy and many of its points of reference require further checking. It appears to us that many of the schizophrenic patient's psychological reactions to his physical and social environment are secondary to a breakdown in his cognitive functions which progressively alienates him from his environment. We have presented evidence which indicates that the schizophrenic patient is abnormally vulnerable to distraction by environmental stimuli. It would also appear that he has particular difficulty in integrating information simultaneously from different sensory channels. The patient's deficit in selective attention has a direct effect on his immediate memory and this would appear to be a primary cause of the pronounced difficulty in communication which is so characteristic of the schizophrenic patient. As a result of the primary breakdown, the patient, when listening to another person speaking, has to attend consciously with deliberation to each unit of information as it is presented. Because of the time taken to assimilate information in this way, sequences of verbal information are particularly difficult for him to cope with. The following comment from one of our patients directly illustrates the subjective aspects of this difficulty: 'I've to pay all my attention to people when they are speaking, otherwise I get all mixed up and don't understand them. I have to think what the words mean. You get all kinds of different thoughts in your head as a result of just one word. For a short time I can concentrate but then a whole sentence I find I haven't taken in . . . You've got to find out the meaning of the sentence. I've to search carefully.' It is in such circumstances that the non-verbal aspects of communication assume great importance. The observer's actions, gestures, mannerisms, facial expression, tone and pitch of voice, may all be utilized by the patient in his attempt to communicate adequately. As one of our patients declared – 'I've got to see somebody to carry on a conversation. It doesn't make sense what they say . . . You read it in their faces what they say.'

It seems probable, therefore, that the actual environmental conditions prevailing at any particular time will have a profound bearing on the patient's current symptomatology and behaviour. From what our patients have told us and from their behaviour in a test situation, it would seem that they are likely to be at a disadvantage in large, noisy wards where there is much irregular activity and where their senses are being bombarded simultaneously by multiple stimuli. In these circumstances, symptoms such as hallucinations, withdrawal, or catatonic behaviour, appear more likely to emerge. Perhaps the most trying source of perceptual overloading of the schizophrenic patient occurs when he has to communicate verbally with a number of people, as in the 'cocktail party' situation.

It is perhaps a truism to say that, in the individual treatment of the schizophrenic patient, one of the main aims is to establish better communication with him. It has been argued often that a better understanding of the current transference relationship and other interpersonal factors will facilitate this and lead to an improvement in the patient's perceptual and cognitive performance. While this may be true, we would argue that the reverse is equally important, in that an understanding of the basic perceptual and cognitive difficulties with which the schizophrenic patient is faced leads to an establishment of better communication and facilitates the development of a good relationship with the therapist. We have found that many schizophrenic patients who are initially withdrawn and uncommunicative are encouraged to speak more freely and to relate themselves more easily to the interviewer by their realization that the basic difficulties which they experience are appreciated and understood.

An understanding of the restrictions imposed on the schizophrenic patient allows one to offer a few simple and practical suggestions which we have found ourselves to be of assistance in interviewing schizophrenic patients. First of all, the arrangement and contents of the interviewing room are kept constant, since the patients are perceptually so sensitive to environmental changes, even to the dress and appearance of the therapist. The interview is conducted with the patient and the therapist sitting squarely face to face, the patient being in a position where he can easily see everything around him, and where he can see the therapist's face and expression clearly. This facilitates the purely physiognomic aspects of communication which can, to some extent, offset the verbal difficulty. All extraneous sources of stimulation inside and outside the room should be reduced as much as possible. Even the hum of the tape-recorder used to record the interview proved to be a frequent source of disturbance reported by patients. The therapist should remain relatively immobile and restrict his actions or gestures unless these are used to transmit meaning. The interview need not become too mechanical or rigid, but it is important to avoid 'irrelevant' movements while attempting to communicate verbally with the patient. The patient should not be left to initiate communication, but his spontaneous verbal responses should be encouraged by providing him with suitable verbal stimuli. Verbal communication itself should be limited, using well-defined items or ideas, and illustrated more by gesture. Verbal information may be more effectively transmitted if it is delivered at a slow, steady rate with scanning of phrases. Abstract words or ideas should be avoided. Where the communication does become more abstract, which is probably inevitable, then the patient must be allowed sufficient time to refer to his own memories and respond without the therapist's interjecting new verbal or other stimuli into the patient's perceptual system, thereby disrupting his own mental activity. The essential requirement in verbal communication is to take the content of what one intends to convey and alter it in such a way that it more readily accommodates to the patient's altered mode of perception. This involves presenting him with small, easily retained, isolated units of meaning which are structured so that they stand out in sharp contrast to the general perceptual background.

CONCLUSIONS

In concluding this account of some experimental investigations of schizophrenia, I should like to re-emphasize the point that our experimental studies have been founded initially on clinical observation. The validity and usefulness of the findings are thus dependent upon the skill and accuracy with which these initial observations were made. The background of our ideas upon which our experimental studies have been built, lies in intensive clinical observation of schizophrenic patients. It was this initial period of study of individual schizophrenic patients and observation of their interactions in groups, which eventually led us to develop the hypotheses which we were subsequently able to subject to experimental verification. We are often asked how we were able to gain the co-operation of these patients in the many experiments in which they have taken part. The answer here again lies in the initial relationship established with the patient before testing. Each of the patients who have taken part in our work had been interviewed on numerous occasions before he was asked to perform any tests. These interviews allowed us not only to collect a great deal of clinical information about the patient, but also to develop a good relationship with the individual patient before the experimental work was started. In the absence of this relationship it is doubtful whether many of the patients would have been sufficiently motivated to co-operate in the long hours of testing involved.

Earlier in this volume Dr Freeman has rightly commented that experimental studies of patients rarely help the clinician in his handling
and treatment of the individual patient. In this discussion we have
attempted to indicate how experimentally derived findings may in fact
have some relevance to the therapeutic handling of the patient. This is,
however, not the main purpose of experimental inquiries of the type
we have described. The rational and effective treatment of any condition depends a great deal on our knowledge of the aetiology of the
condition in question. In the case of schizophrenia, it seems fairly obvious that we are dealing with a very heterogeneous sample of patients
and that we are unlikely to find a single aetiology or a single effective
treatment. An adequate system of classification of the schizophrenias
is thus perhaps our first requirement. What little we have learned of the
aetiology of the so-called functional psychoses strongly suggests that
the term functional is misleading and that we are dealing here with an
organic psychosis. This viewpoint has caused some psychiatrists to
feel that the clinician's future contribution in this field must be slight,
and that the key to the aetiology of schizophrenia will one day be
provided by the biochemist and the physiologist. On the contrary, it
would seem that further progress must depend on the reliability and
validity of the clinical diagnosis and classification of schizophrenia.
In reviewing our current knowledge of the physiopathology of schizophrenia, Tait (1958) concluded: ' . . . I do not personally believe that
one single biochemical answer to what we call schizophrenia will be
found. The biochemist and the electro-physiologist are more likely
to give us a set of answers, and I could wish we were in a position to
give them a set of questions which were equally precise and clearly
defined. I feel that we must exploit old or develop new methods of
defining and measuring our schizophrenic states.' More recently Slater
& Beard (1963), reporting on their comparative study of schizophrenia
and epileptic psychosis, concluded: 'One might take the view that with
schizophrenia we are now approaching the stage of understanding
which was reached half a century ago with epilepsy. It was customary
then to classify the epilepsies into ideopathic and symptomatic types,
and in the latter case to specify the underlying condition of which the
epilepsy was symptomatic. This rather primitive stage in subclassifica-
tion may now become possible in the syndrome we call schizophrenia.
Very likely the bulk of the cases so diagnosed will prove to be "idio-
pathic", with genetic factors responsible for the specificities. But
round this nucleus we would aim to define, with increasing precision,

groups of cases in which the schizophrenia-like psychosis was traceable to known processes.' Perhaps, then, the main contribution which experimental psychology can make to the problem of schizophrenia is in increasing the precision of this process of clinical delineation by producing reasonably objective and reliable means of assessing the different changes in mental function which occur in different forms of the psychosis.

CHAPTER 10

The Psycho-analytic Treatment
of the Psychoses

The application of psycho-analytic methodology to the treatment of the major mental disorders is nowadays no longer regarded as an experimental or tentative procedure in many of the state hospitals in the United States. The resident medical staff feel that their training is being neglected if their work with disturbed patients is not supervised by a psycho-analyst. This is part of the therapeutic armamentarium with which they expect to be equipped, and they regard themselves as being inadequately trained if they have not been taught the basic principles of the psychotherapy of the psychoses.

It would, of course, be a strange reflection if it were not the case that, forty years after the initial work of Federn, a well-proved technique had not been developed. It is of some interest to note, however, that there is still a tendency to regard such work as pioneering, as something uncertain, ill-defined, and vague. This view, widely held in some places, is an interesting one, particularly when one considers the frequency with which a third-year resident already has a therapeutic success in such a venture under his belt. This is quite apart from the nowadays quite formidable literature on the subject, varying from Paul Federn's initial descriptions of the work, to the more recent writings of Harold F. Searles.

It would be easy to dismiss the tenacity with which this view is held, as a manifestation of a somewhat generalized, unconscious resistance, which tends to keep blanketed the at times terrifying primary processes of mentation. Another view of the situation is to appreciate that the work is arduous, difficult, frequently disappointing, anxiety-provoking, and, in particular, time-consuming. Here one runs into the economic problem, for five years or so of inpatient psychotherapy is an expensive business, regardless of whether the cost is met by the patient's family or by a National Health Service.

A basic belief held in Chestnut Lodge is that one cannot really expect a psychotherapist to begin to function effectively until he has been working in this field for a minimum of three years. In my own view, this estimate is a minimal one. Because of these factors, then, although it may be true that people tend to shrink away from the work because of psychological resistance, there are serious economic and training problems which interfere with the intent of individuals who are na- tively or through the benefit of personal analysis able to overcome the difficulty due to resistance. With all of this in mind, I should like to address myself to what I have learned in the ten years in which I have worked as a psycho-analyst on the staff of Chestnut Lodge.

THE MILIEU

The milieu within which the psycho-analytic psychotherapy of psycho- tic patients proceeds must have special provisions which are unnecessary in the treatment of the neuroses. Special problems of patient administra- tion arise which cannot be dealt with by the psychotherapist. It is impor- tant to remember that the prognosis of a patient undergoing analysis is not the prognosis of an individual but the prognosis of a therapeutic relationship, and the administrator who is responsible for making judge- ments regarding an analytic patient must constantly have in mind the nature of the therapeutic process operating between the particular therapist and his particular patient.

For a period I worked as consultant in psycho-analysis at a state hospital. It was held there that no difference existed between the patient who was in psychotherapy and the patient who was not. On two occasions a discharge conference was held when the patients were in a state of social recovery. In both instances the patient was discharged without consultation with the therapist. The reactions of the therapists in question made it clear to the hospital staff that the therapeutic relationship should have been taken into account. In one of the situ- ations there were ominous overtones because both therapist and super- visor were of the opinion that the social recovery, satisfactory from the point of view of a hospital seeking merely this, represented in the therapeutic situation the patient's defence against suicidal preoccupations based on the depressive fear that she would destroy her therapist as she felt she had done with everyone whom she had previously loved.

A means of dealing with such a difficulty is to combine the functions of therapist and administrator. This is, of course, feasible in a situation where the therapy takes a counselling and even a directive mode. For the more sophisticated therapist, however, who is concerned with the analysis of subtler manifestations of the patient's narcissistic transference, the maintenance of a more neutral position is imperative. This is achieved in Chestnut Lodge by dividing the functions so that the administrator is responsible for general hospital living, while the therapist attends to treatment. In this situation the therapist is free to consider the all-important symbolic overtones of the patient's productions. To quote Searles (1963): 'If to use a simple example, both therapeutic and administrative functions were the responsibility of a single physician that physician would find it especially hard to discern, in a patient's insistent demands to "move out", a subtle symbolic meaning which the patient is unable to formulate as such in his own mind, namely a plea for help in "moving out" of his shell, out of his isolation *vis-à-vis* his fellow men.'

All of this does not mean, however, that skills and knowledge acquired by an administrative physician elsewhere may not be utilized in a psycho-analytic hospital. All that is required of him is to remember that he is dealing with patients in analysis, and that estimates must be made with due attention to the state of the analytic process. For example, some physicians develop in their wards highly refined and sophisticated group processes involving patient government, in the course of which the administrator delegates to the group considerable decision-making responsibilities. Such an administrator must remember the nature of responsibility, for one can only delegate that authority which one actually has.

It is a cardinal rule of psycho-analytic administration that when a patient is protectively restricted for behaviour which imperils him in some way, then that protective curtailment of his activity must be maintained until the patient has had an opportunity to explore his motivation with his therapist so that the tendency to repeat the behaviour has been reduced. During such a period, the administrator does not have the authority to extend the patient's privileges and, accordingly, cannot delegate such authority to the patient-government process. Once he has been notified by the therapist that some resolution of the difficulty has occurred, he is free to take that action which in his clinical judgement is best for the patient.

Another difference between psycho-analytically oriented administration and standard mental hospital practice is to be seen on the occasion of visits from the family. So far from feeling that it would be pleasant for the family to have an unsupervised meal outside the hospital the psycho-analytic administrator will be more apt to increase restrictions on the patient in view of his belief that inherent in the family constellation are those pathogenic interpersonal factors which produced the patient's illness. Accordingly, the occasions of family visits are ones that require increased alertness on the part of the staff to the possibility of the repetition of manifestations of the original difficulty.

Some years ago a psycho-analyst in Chestnut Lodge went to see a powerful paranoid individual who was capable of outbursts of murderous rage. The patient's parents were in the ward visiting at the time. The patient launched a physical attack on the therapist who dodged quickly to the other side of the patient's bed. As the patient ran around to seize him the therapist shouted, 'Don't you realize you do this every time your parents visit?' The patient stopped dead in his tracks and sat down on the bed, saying in a horrified voice, 'My God — you're right — so I do.'

Such considerations, of course, apply merely to the simplest and most fundamental implications of the application of the psychoanalytic method. They can be underlined and emphasized over and over again by illustrations upon which the broad, basic principles are founded. A therapist with a year's experience behind him will be well aware of the patient's reaction to hours which have been missed by the therapist. The separation anxiety which flares up on such occasions may or may not be adequately dealt with in the psycho-analytic process. Accordingly, a psycho-analytic administrator will regard times when the therapist is absent on vacation as the worst possible occasion to regard favourably a request for a visit home.

It is only too easy for the unskilled to listen sympathetically to such requests as the following: 'But doctor, this is the best possible time for me to go home. My therapist is away on vacation himself. I will not be missing my real treatment since he is not here to give it to me. The hospital is of no value to me while he is absent. You must surely see my point, for is not psycho-analysis the cornerstone of treatment in this hospital?' Since psycho-analysis *is* the cornerstone of the psycho-analytic administrator's programme, he must at once say 'no' to such a request because of his awareness of the patient's increased anxiety over the therapist's absence, and despite his sympathy for the distress produced by this inevitable part of the patient's progress toward recovery.

This is, of course, no hard-and-fast rule, for it may well be that the patient is at a point in psycho-analytic treatment where the highly personal nature of separation anxiety has been adequately investigated and the therapist can reassure the administrator that in this particular case such a decision can safely be made. Such decisions are in fact risky in the interpersonal sense, for the administrator who makes them casually may earn for himself the extreme disapproval of a therapist who has worked with a patient for six to seven years if he is faced with the fact that a junior administrator has made a snap decision, ignoring basic psycho-analytic principles, and allowed the patient home. The therapist of the psychoses is not at his peak for a very long period. Most know this, and are apt to be somewhat sensitive should one-sixth of their professional life during this period be casually cast on one side in the name of being nice.

Such 'maladministration' is fortunately uncommon, and now I should like to refer to another and more highly skilled area of administration which requires brief consideration — namely, the truly individual and psycho-analytic administration of the individual case. This particular area is one which demands a special skill, theoretical knowledge, and formulative ability on the part of the administrator. I do not mean by this some special, highly abstractive skill, for the factors involved in the formulation often escape attention.[1]

The patient was involved in a paranoidly defended symbiotic relationship with her mother, and consequently in the transference with the therapist. Many defence mechanisms were naturally operating that successfully repressed all cognizance of such factors. The symptomatic manifestation of this repression showed in a rationally defended preference for anything that was in any way connected with the patient's home state of California. Anything from California was good, superior, morally finer than anything in Maryland. Following a discussion of the therapeutic problem with the therapist, the administrator made an administrative shift which led to a rapid resolution of the defence.

The manoeuvre was marvellous in its simplicity, for all that the

[1] I am indebted to Dr S. Sheila Hafter for permission to use the following administrative example in which she was the administrator and I was the therapist.

administrator did was to give the patient a roommate whose personal habits, including exhibitionist masturbatory tendencies, were somewhat difficult for a lady to tolerate. When the patient had ventilated most forcibly her annoyance with this individual, the therapist was finally able to say, 'I am surprised to hear from you that you find it so difficult to share a room with a fellow Californian.' This was the end of the particular defence which had proved so troublesome and, in my opinion, one truly deft application of psycho-analytic finesse shortened treatment by many months, for the symbiotic relationship with the hospital, and with the therapist in particular, then came under psycho-analytic scrutiny and led to a freeing of mental energy as the patient began to examine the transference nature of this relationship, *vis-à-vis* her mother.

Of course, one cannot always expect this kind of insight, from which springs the ability to take a simple action having such marked effect. One can always work with the patient for an extra year in the hope of a similar result, but such manoeuvres can be confidently anticipated when the administrator is in his or her own right a well-trained therapist and one whose relationship with the analyst enables such formulations to be made. Just as such talented administration can further the psycho-analytic process, so unskilled management can impede it. A therapist has no right to expect the kind of manoeuvre described which fortifies the therapeutic process. He is entitled, however, to demand adherence to the basic concepts previously outlined. *Further research and investigation into the administration of the psychotic patient in analysis is, in my opinion, the most promising route to the abbreviation of the protracted course of treatment which at this point is the major obstacle in the way of a more generalized application of psychotherapy to the psychoses.* Due attention should be given to the personality and needs of individuals who in an early stage of their training are capable of the kind of administrative manoeuvre carried out by the administrator already mentioned. It is from them that we may learn shortcuts which will enable our methodology to be more readily applied.

As an administrator with some years of experience in this field, I do not wish to be misunderstood. Milieu management and social recovery are a poor substitute for a satisfactory analytic result of treatment because of which a disturbed individual never requires to see a psychiatrist again except, perhaps, in a social setting. One cannot divorce theory from practice, and I should like to make a plea for the theoretically sound, yet highly ingenious psycho-analytic administrator whose talents, when combined with those of a well-trained and well-supervised psycho-analyst, can lead to that most satisfactory of all medical interventions, namely, the recovery of a profoundly disturbed psychotic individual.

PSYCHO-ANALYTIC MANAGEMENT

The psycho-analytic management of psychotic patients falls within the prerogative of the analyst. Confusion between psycho-analytic management and psycho-analytic administration frequently leads to difficulty. Some years ago an analyst in Chestnut Lodge complained to an administrator that a patient was scribbling on his door. The administrator asked whether the scribbling was on the inside or the outside of the office door. On being told that the scribbling was on the inside of the door, the administrator responded, 'Inside the door is therapy, outside the door is administration. Since the scribbling is inside the door, that is a therapeutic and not an administrative problem. Take it up with your patient yourself, for that is your business.' Although this example tends to caricature the difference, it is none the less valid, for what goes on in the hour is strictly the analyst's business, even if he may invite administrative assistance.

In the management of psychotic patients it is important to recognize that a disturbed individual may be so disorganized that he cannot comply with the basic rules of psycho-analysis. The golden rule of the treatment, as applied to neurotic patients, is that the patient should say whatever comes into his mind. Implicit in this statement, however, is a multiplicity of other rules, such as the demand that the patient should appear on time, lie down, and say whatever comes to mind. Beyond this again are those which state that the patient will not urinate or defecate on the office floor. Above and beyond all this, of course, are such simple considerations as the fact that the patient is expected not to smash up the office furniture or throw side tables through the windows. Let us be clear that no psychic structure or impulse control can be confidently expected from people suffering from psychotic illnesses by the very definition of the nature of the disorder itself.

As has already been indicated, psycho-analytic management refers to those fundamental rules of behaviour during the psycho-analytic session which are necessary for the maintenance of the psycho-analytic relationship. For those analysts who are accustomed to a private practice dealing predominantly with minor mental disorders, many of these rules remain tacit throughout the entire treatment programme. No such unspoken assumptions may be made in the treatment of some of our more disordered patients. For an adequate psycho-analytic programme to be maintained, both parties involved in the transaction must survive. The application of psycho-analytic principles to a corpse is clearly as unsatisfactory as to attempt to imagine that a dead psycho-analyst will be of much value to the analysand. The cardinal principle, then, of psycho-analytic management is to ensure the maintenance and continuation of the treatment programme. It is mandatory that the analyst should quite explicitly take all such steps as are necessary to this end and that these steps should be spelled out clearly and openly to the patient in the hope that the undamaged aspect of the ego will grasp the intent, regardless of the psychotic interpretations which are placed upon them.

If there can be a rule about the difficulties implicit in the therapy of the psychoses it should be that the analyst takes a conservative view in all situations, for one can always apologize if one has been over-cautious in the name of treatment, whereas one may not have the opportunity if one has been over-confident. The other cardinal rule is honesty. One should not pretend to some other motive when one does not wish to see one's patient. Should the analyst feel that it is necessary to place the patient in physical restraint, such as a wet sheet pack, he should make it clear why. A simple statement will suffice. 'I have found your manner menacing and accordingly have given orders that you should be in a pack. First of all, I have no wish to be injured while working and, secondly, I find that I cannot function effectively as your analyst when I am alarmed for my own safety.' One of my colleagues put the position in a more colourful way when he stated, 'Listen, friend, I am here to earn my living, not the Order of the Purple Heart.'

The survival of the analytical relationship requires not merely the actual survival of the analyst, but actually as great a degree of comfort for him as is feasible in a relationship which is inevitably disturbed. The therapist who is subject to too great stress in the course of his work will in some way or other withdraw from the relationship. This phenomenon has been well illustrated in two papers by Farber (1958, 1963). The difficult countertransference aspects of the work are also well illustrated in the writings of Harold Searles.

The welfare of the patient is, in the same fundamental sense, of maximum importance in the psychotherapeutic venture. Treatment cannot continue with a patient who has died by his own hand and treatment goes badly with a patient whose hours are interrupted for a variety of reasons, varying from deliberate self-destructive activities to avoidance of psycho-analytic sessions. The analyst should not hesitate to interdict such behaviour, taking the necessary action in the name of the preservation of the relationship. A not untypical destructive act against the maintenance of treatment by patients who find difficulty in expressing their antagonism and dissatisfaction with the work is to communicate with their family in such a way as to ensure family intervention and even transfer to another hospital. Such patients, when talking with their analysts, frequently shake their heads sadly over the family's irruption into the treatment situation and may even attempt to persuade the analyst that he is witnessing another piece of the family's pathology which was causal in the development of the patient's illness. The more experienced analyst will recognize the mutuality of such family interaction and draw the patient's attention to it with the warning that the patient can, in fact, terminate treatment by these methods if he wishes to. It is only by bringing such material at once into focus that such behaviour can be prevented.

At all times, of course, one is dependent to some extent on the self-reflective and collaborative aspect of the patient's ego. At no point should one lose sight of this, for the patient also has some responsibility for seeking his own recovery, and the analyst who loses sight of this burdens himself with too great a degree of responsibility, however experienced and skilful he may be. He is only partly responsible for a therapeutic success. The true success belongs to the patient who has been able to utilize the psycho-analyst's technical skill. The same applies to therapeutic failure, for the analyst again can only be responsible for exercising that degree of professional skill which is in accordance with his training. There are two features of this work which are worthwhile recording. If, for example, one notes that one is being required to produce more than one ordinarily does, one should suspect that one is being required to be omnipotent. Should these demands lead to an ignoring of the boundaries between management and administration and, in particular, if one finds oneself tempted to correct the administrator too often, then something is being missed in treatment and one is, most probably, collaborating with one's patient in avoiding his extreme narcissistic disappointment and rage, which are an essential part of the original narcissistic injury that must, of course, unfold in the transference where it can be adequately analysed.

Supervision

A part of the psycho-analytic management that must never be under-estimated is the function of supervision. In the course of the psycho-analysis of narcissism the development of the transference psychosis is usually extremely intense and may totally swamp the self-reflective aspects of the ego. At such times the burden upon the analyst is intense and the problem is aggravated by the fact that at these very times the analyst's countertransference is particularly strong. The interplay of such forces in the interpersonal relationship can only too easily lead to a narcissistic block, a kind of interlocking which produces a therapeutic impasse. This possibility must never be ignored, even with the most experienced and skilled analysts. One can go so far as to say that the more skilled, the more experienced the analyst, the more apt he him-self will be to seek supervision and the more apt he will be to listen carefully to a dispassionate voice, uninvolved in the painful bind, which can be so useful in helping him and the patient to find some objectivity in their relationship again.

Supervision is perhaps the most difficult technically of all the tasks discussed so far, for it is necessary for the supervisor to be well ac-quainted with the various vicissitudes of the narcissistic transference. I hope that later in this chapter the technicalities of the management of such extremely difficult relationships will become more explicit.

General Consideration

In a brief review such as the one contained in this chapter, it is impos-sible to cover adequately the complexities of either psycho-analytic administration or analytic management. Only a brief reference has been made to the complexities of the interplay between family and patient, implicit within which are the pathogenic factors which have produced as its resolution the current situation that the analyst is seeking to alter — namely, one family member is in hospital diagnosed as suffering from a major mental disorder. Whether the analyst likes it or not, he is a participant in this situation and he should at no time allow himself to be deceived about this, for his pretence to analytic neutrality may veritably be an avoidance of the very forces he is seeking to combat. The saddest lesson I had to learn in the course of my work in Chestnut Lodge was a somewhat painful one, namely, the interruption of my very best work, because I did not take into account those forces within the family which had produced the clinical state in the patient. One moment of carelessness destroyed the entire therapeutic venture.

I should like, quite briefly, to illustrate my point with this sad error. The patient was a very disturbed man who had, at the time of the initial therapeutic intervention, been suffering from a condition best described as Bell's Mania. The intervention had prevented the death of the patient and ten months later the therapist was dealing with those primitive elements of the psychogenesis which were the cornerstone of a narcissistic illness. At about this time, the patient's mother visited the hospital and the therapist, with the patient's knowledge, interviewed the lady in question. In a moment of therapeutic enthusiasm he confided in the mother his dim grasp of her plight many years before. As a result of his comments he received evidence from her to support the hypothesis upon which his work was based. Unfortunately, he ignored the fact that such an exchange between himself and the patient's mother left the patient's father with the alternative of facing his own pathology or obscuring it by an expression of dissatisfaction with his son's current clinical state. Shortly afterwards, the father, a physician, visited the hospital accompanied by his brother, a distinguished professor from a leading university. The brother was present, of course, to add a stamp of medical approval to the father's preordained conclusion. The patient was transferred from the hospital, and consequently from the therapist's care, in the face of the brother's opposition to such a move.

Ordinarily, the position of the analyst in dealing with the minor neuroses is clear cut, for the reporting of progress in the treatment is the responsibility of the patient. This, of course, cannot be the case with the hospitalized patient, who may, in fact, be mute. Often the administrative physician can deal with such situations, but at times only the intervention of the analyst, through personal interview with the relatives, can protect the treatment situation. As a result of my experiences in such situations, I have developed a series of broad rules which I follow. First, I prefer to see relatives only in the presence of the patient. Second, such interviews are normally held on the instigation of the patient. Third, I reserve at all times the right to be arbitrary, *vis-à-vis* the patient, when I feel that such an interview with or without the patient is imperative for the maintenance of the analysis. At such a point, however, the analyst should take cognizance of the possibility that his judgement may be in error, not merely in instituting the interview, but also in the management of the content of that interview, as is so sadly apparent in the example mentioned in the previous paragraph.

The best insurance the analyst can take against such errors of judgement is, in my opinion, the utilization of another analyst as supervisor, either formally or informally. One of my private observations regarding the work of Dr Harold F. Searles was that this analyst missed no opportunity, formal or informal, of expounding the problems with which he was faced in the course of his therapeutic work.

THE PSYCHO-ANALYTIC TREATMENT OF PSYCHOSES

In the consideration of psychotic states, I propose to restrict myself to those conditions which, in my opinion, belong within the psychogenetic classification of oral disorders. I would not wish to imply by this that a specific trauma occurs within a definitely delimited period of childhood development, but merely that a characteristic and ongoing pathological interaction with family members, and with the mother in particular, occurred at a sufficiently early age to influence the most basic positing of human characterology. The term 'ongoing' is not to be ignored, for, in my experience, the interaction between mother and fifty-year-old offspring can be still as active as it was in the first year of life.

This formulation does not imply an aetiological hypothesis. Factors other than psychological ones may be at work in the production of psychotic reactions. A one-sided view that overemphasizes the role of the psychological factor can lead easily into unwarranted assumptions such as that of the schizophrenogenic mother. Should a hypermotile child be born to a mother who is concerned greatly with tidiness and control, the seeds of trouble are clearly already there. Does one seek, then, pathology in the mother's minor obsessionalism or in the constitutional givens of hypermotility? These are unanswered questions. From the point of view of the therapist, however, the questions are viewed from a different position, for he is a physician who hopes merely, like Paré, to bandage the wounds of his patient, that God may heal him. Accordingly, he must take cognizance of such psychopathology as is apparent in the patient in the hope of being able to use his technical knowledge to further the latter's welfare.

The treatment of narcissistic disorders is not a simple matter, by virtue of the extraordinary complexity of the manifestations of orality, especially when the picture is further complicated by the presence of regressive and non-regressive features. For the purpose of supplying some unifying theme to this short account of the treatment of such abnormal states, discussion will be limited predominantly to references to the transference and its management in the various disorders.

AUTISM

This clinical condition was originally described by Kanner (1949) as one occurring in children. In his view, the condition is one in which the children are often intelligent, are immobile of facies, and are more interested in objects than in people; their speech, when they do speak, is characterized by concreteness and by errors in the use of pronouns. When discussing a paper concerning the treatment of an adult patient, Kanner commented that he had often wondered what happened to autistic children and now he knew — they became autistic adults (Darr & Worden, 1951).

In the past ten years Margaret Mahler (1952, 1958) has refined this concept further by describing two main clinical categories of autism: first, true autism; and, second, symbiotic autism. In the first category the power of speech is little, if at all, developed and in psychogenetic terms can be likened to a very early stage of orality characterized by narcissism, autistic mentation, minimal frustration tolerance, and an ability to relate only to need-satisfying objects (Freud, A., 1952) of the most elemental type. The symbiotic group may have highly developed powers of speech and rather more complex powers of mentation, with the beginnings of secondary processes, but the object-relatedness is still characterized by a seeking for a need-satisfying object.

My experience of such patients is limited, since I have worked with only one patient in the first category and two in the second. On the basis of these three experiences of long and intensive therapy, plus some supervisory and consultative involvement with physicians treating patients in this clinical category, I have reached the conclusion that the condition of autism is best regarded as a state of true psychogenetic arrest and, accordingly, as a state quite different from the schizophrenias, in which more highly differentiated processes can be observed and in which regression plays so marked a part.

In the process of working with such patients, the writings of Searles (1960) on the non-human environment are of considerable value. It is startling and disconcerting for the therapist to find himself viewed simply as nutrition of some sort. One of my patients did not distinguish me from the glass of apple juice which he was often given during a therapeutic session. The other two regarded me similarly. One made little differentiation between his therapeutic hour and the cigarettes he was allowed to smoke during the session. The third was not interested in differentiating between the therapist and his 'little car'. Her main interest during the hour was to go for a drive in that little car. I have encountered other therapists who had similar difficulty in accepting the fact that they were simply a candybar.

Recognition of the state of object-relatedness is the crux of the management of the transference, and one must build upon these simple, biological givens if one wishes to progress even a little towards psychological maturity. Utilizing the analytical model as a constant guide and check, and keeping in mind such basic concepts as the fact that frustration tends towards structure, while at the same time never ignoring Sullivan's emphasis on the learning process, one can make some steps towards psychological maturation. For example, on one occasion the therapist came to the unit in which lived the patient who regarded him as part of his car. She was bad-tempered, upset, and had a bruise on her face. When he asked about the injury, the patient would not respond and merely asked to go for a ride in the little car to a place where she knew she could get some coffee. Accordingly, they went over together to his office, near which stood his car. When she wished to get into his car, the therapist insisted on going into his office. When she repeated her demand to go for the drive and the coffee, she was told, 'We can go for the drive and the coffee when you have told me how your face became bruised.' After some fussing and a brief demonstration of her capacity to throw a temper-tantrum, the patient finally gave a full account of the incident, which made it clear that she had not been the object of unnecessary violence by the staff, but had bumped her face at a time when they were attempting to control one of her temper-tantrums.

It was my observation that the constant use of my awareness of the state of the object-relatedness led to a gradual increase in the manifestations of psychic structure in the patient and a steady improvement in the handling of frustration. A reasonable limited goal of therapy at such stages is to aim for the development of ambivalence so that, with the introjection of an ambivalently viewed object, there will be a marked increase in psychic structure and the beginnings of development of object constancy.

If the analytic model is not kept before one during such work, the therapist can readily deceive himself regarding the mental state, particularly with those patients who belong in the symbiotic category. At this point it is important to stress that it is the nature of the transference which must always be kept in mind. The following example illustrates this point. The therapist had been delighted with the success of some of his interpretations in such a case. It finally dawned upon him that perhaps he was revelling in the pleasures of the 'white island of motherhood', the Nirvana State of Barbara Low, for he knew only too well that the omniscience of giving the ever perfect, ever correctly timed interpretation was indeed something which he could not achieve. The patient had been complaining of something which he called 'the horrible feeling', a condition involving perceptual disturbances and a generalized discomfort best viewed in Mahler's terms as organismic distress.

It appeared from his account of 'the horrible feeling' that it occurred at a different time on the days when the therapist saw the patient, as compared with those days when there was no analytic hour. A transference and interpersonal interpretation was offered and was greeted with confirmatory data from the patient. Further attempts at exploration did not get very far. Closer examination of the simple phenomenology revealed that the horrible feeling was not related to the analytic hour but to mealtimes, and the mealtime was different on the days when he saw the analyst from the days when he did not. The horrible feeling was the result of his undifferentiated inability to appreciate the distress of hunger, and this lack of differentiation was reinforced by his environment, which was in itself so disorganized that his mentors sometimes forgot to feed him.

This finding is of importance in terms of the environment's co-operation in the maintenance of the autistic state. However, for the therapist, the transference is, as always, *the factor of cardinal significance.* The patient's confirmation of the analyst's erroneous interpretations was based upon his need to please him, to maintain in him the affective tone that would sustain his role as a need-satisfying object. In more everyday language, all the patient was doing was to keep the therapist in a good mood so that he would be given cigarettes during the next session. This is not a speculative observation, but something which became repeatedly manifest during the four years of this patient's treatment.

Perhaps of some interest theoretically in the treatment of autistic patients is the appearance of mental processes (appropriate verbal communication) which are often regarded as characteristic of later psychogenetic evolution. For example, Bill was an autistic young man who had been in treatment with me four times a week for seven months; he was the individual whose main interest in therapy was focused on his daily ration of cigarettes, about which more will be said later. When I returned from a month's absence on vacation, I was greeted with a series of telephone requests for assistance and advice from the people privately employed by his family to look after him. They were mostly individuals without any special training in the field. As far as they were concerned, the patient was, in some uncanny and awful sort of way, quite out of control.

It transpired that they had tied the patient hand and foot to his bed to control him. I advised them to move the breakable items out of his reach and turn him loose, but in the meantime I sent a well-trained practical nurse from the hospital to look after him for the night. She, incidentally, mothered him a bit, chased everybody else away, and finally tucked him up for the night. The following day when Bill arrived for his hour he was dishevelled, untidy, and unshaven, and walked with a quite grotesque gait. His pelvis seemed tilted at an angle of forty-five degrees so that he hobbled when he tried to walk. In the therapist's office he limped back and forth in this manner, talking in a voice quite incoherent, but full of rage and distress. Finally the therapist, somewhat at a loss to know what to say, commented, 'I gather, Bill, that you have been rather badly hurt.' With that, the patient's bodily contortion disappeared and he sat down and gave an account of the event, venting fully his rage and indignation at the indignity he had suffered and, in particular, complaining to the therapist that he should not have abandoned him in the way he had done.

It is worth of note that the therapist did not, in the confusion of the moment, expect to produce such a marked and dramatic shift in the patient by virtue of his comment. What is important is the loose and primitive nature of the cathexes (primary process) underlying the symptoms – a characteristic not merely of the unconscious but of orality. I have found it useful to remember when dealing with patients in other clinical categories who present conversion and somatic symptoms, that there too there is an oral component, attention to which has rapidly produced resolution of the resistance with considerable freeing of psychic energy.

As was mentioned earlier, the transference with this patient could best be appreciated by watching for evidence of the need-satisfying object in the transference. Its nature, in this case, cannot be appreciated unless one realizes that, with the lack of psychic differentiation, to be deprived of his cigarettes was to be deprived of his mother's milk, the very sustenance of life itself. This showed very clearly in an exchange which also indicates some factors operating in a tape-recorded session. The recording was made by a research worker in another organization with the patient's prior agreement and approval. At the time, the central theme of the therapeutic work centred on memory function. The patient and the therapist would compare notes on what they had eaten since they had last seen each other. At the beginning of the hour, he somewhat tentatively tried to find out what should be discussed. He began with the topic of meals. After telling the therapist that he had had two boiled eggs and some bacon for breakfast, he suddenly made the following comment: 'I have a fear that this tape and this recording might interfere with our work, so I have the feeling that it makes me less tense when we are talking through the tape-recording because it gives me something new to think about.' After talking about the recording, the therapist finally said to him, 'You were saying that you were uneasy that it might interefere with our work in some way,' and he said, 'Well, I figure it might interfere with our work or it might interfere with my cigarettes.' After some further discussion, the therapist said, 'How do you think it might interfere with our work or with your cigarettes, Bill?' He answered, 'Well, they might get the idea that you shouldn't give me the cigarettes, those people, when they are studying us, when they check up on us it might give them the idea that you shouldn't give me cigarettes any more.' Later he said, 'They might criticize you for giving me a cigarette, if you see what I mean.'

The basic reference is to the nature of his relationship to his mother, who, in her desperation, was constantly seeking new professional advice in his management. With each new person, the technique of his rearing varied, so that Bill's suspicion that the therapist would readily allow the rules of his treatment situation to be changed through the influence of some outside person's opinion was firmly and repetitiously rooted in his past experience. There was another side to his attitude to the tape-recording, however, for he saw it as possibly being of some value to him, and he expatiated into the microphone upon the iniquities of various people who had looked after him in the course of his life and who had offended him in some way. It was his openly expressed wish that those influential people who would listen to the tape would take some steps to penalize the sinners whom he had described. This

particular aspect of exhibitionism is an interesting example of the complexity of orality.

Despite all this, one still has to work through the process of separation
from the symbiotic relationship, that terribly disillusioning psychic
weaning from omnipotence and identification with an omnipotent
mother, which is the healthy prototype of the unhealthy, narcissistic
wound, so pathogenic in subsequent mental development. In the case
of Bill, this process took an interesting form, one which has been well
documented as part of narcissism (see Searles, 1959). Bill had told me
in the first year of treatment that he regarded his mother as different
from other mothers. For example, she always acceded to all his
requests. At one time, apparently, he had been allowed to drink beer.
He was never satisfied with one can of beer and he used to nag her for
another and another and another until finally he got sick. He had
confided to me that although he liked this quality in her he also was
scornful of it and regarded her as crazy for being so easy.

In the sessions he referred to the personality of his coloured chauffeur.
He knew I liked this man because he was firm enough in his manner
always to ensure arrival at the office at the stated time. The patient
was chuckling to himself a great deal and asked if I thought that
Tom (the chauffeur) was funny because of his firmness. This led
on during these hours to his inquiring whether or not Tom was different from other people. Apparently, in his opinion, Tom was different
from all the other chauffeurs, and at that point I began to catch on that
Tom was a different sort of mother, namely, a crazy one. Occasionally
he would meditate and chuckle to himself and was inclined to ignore
me. Occasionally he would admit that he was laughing to himself
about something I had said. Before long, the tenor of his questions was
directed along a line which may be anticipated. Although superficially
he seemed to be complimenting me, he was trying to nudge me out on
a limb where I was the world's only psychotherapist, and in any case if
I was not the world's only psychotherapist then I was a pretty unusual
one because I didn't use drugs. But even if others didn't use drugs, then
surely I was the only one who was so strict about the rules of treatment.
About this time I heard from Bill's home that they all thought I was
the daftest doctor permitted to practise in the length and breadth of
the country. The patient had done a fine job of persuading them of
this. However, as I am not nearly so nice or so tolerant a person as the
mother, the next time he and I met, the patient was seriously confronted
with some of his activities. This was sharpened by the fact that the

clinical director of the hospital had drawn my attention to a variety of ways in which Bill was making a nuisance of himself. What eventually emerged was the fact that he had quite consciously been preoccupied with the idea that I was crazy and had been seeking to prove it.

It was during this period, which lasted for some time, that the patient first began to distinguish between his wishes and those of the therapist and to appreciate that neither was omnipotent. For the first time he became clearly and freely able to express strongly hostile ideas without feeling that a disaster would occur. With this establishment of ambivalence, a most important structural psychic change occurred, as is demonstrated by the following clinical example from that time. He was looking fed up and depressed when he came into the office and he very quickly let me know that he was angry. It was a Monday hour and he had not been seen since the previous Friday, so I was at a loss when I was told something which the patient had frequently said before, namely, that I often said things that hurt his feelings. He had given no such indication on the Friday, and when this was raised with him, with the intention of exploring the reason for withholding such important data, the patient said, 'That is not what I mean, John. It was in my home that I got mad with you. I was on my way to beg some cigarettes and I suddenly remembered you telling me that, by doing this, I annoyed people, and might lose all my new privileges. I could even see you saying it when I thought of it and I was very mad with you for saying that.' This indication of a differentiated superego was a source of great gratification to me, particularly when Bill went on to say that this hurtful remark from the installed superego figure had, in fact, delayed his seeking immediate gratification, for he had not gone for the cigarettes, had not got into trouble, but instead had come back in accordance with the good old analytic rule and had raised Cain with his therapist.

Such a differentiation between the self and the not-self in the psychic structure opens the way for very considerable development. Having recognized the other person as one capable of saying 'No' (of being, in Fairbairn's (1952) terms, a frustrating object), the individual is also freed to say 'no' himself and thus affirm himself as a separate entity. This *affirmative no*, as I prefer to call it, is a most important event in psychogenesis, which, nonetheless, in the context of pathology, can produce troublesome manifestations varying from negativism, on the one hand, to the negative, therapeutic reaction, on the other. These features will receive attention as we proceed to a consideration of the transference in other narcissistic disorders.

Some brief mention has to be made of my countertransference experiences with autistic patients, to the unconscious aspects of my relationship with them. Perhaps the most noteworthy feature of psychotherapeutic work in autistic states is its undramatic quality. Things are experienced in a somewhat muted tone, apart from the odd occasion when the patient's generalized distress leads to a temper-tantrum, which can be startling and has been described by Ferster (1961) as atavistic behaviour. For the therapist with some experience of the rage of a schizophrenic patient, these outbursts have a non-threatening and muted quality, which, in my experience, is inherent in its undifferentiated and undirected quality.

On the conscious level, the main negative reaction takes the form of a kind of dull boredom, quite different, subjectively, from the apathy or somnolent detachment which sometimes appears in the work with the other narcissistic states. At times the therapist has difficulty explaining to himself the reason for his continued interest in the work. Similarly, the satisfactions and pleasures are marked by the same undifferentiated quality. When they are tracked down, they are sometimes of a somewhat primitive nature. For example, in the case of one female patient, I used to speak rather jocularly of her importance to me, because she was an extra on my hospital caseload for which I received additional pay. In an informal supervisory situation, I became aware that this jocular manner concealed some considerable anxiety on my part about this subject, for, in fact, the money was extremely important and dominated my attitude to an extent that I felt to be unprofessional.

Examination of this phenomenon produced some interesting data. When I originally started work with this patient I was in the middle of my own analytic training, was somewhat short of funds, but was too busy even to notice it. The extra income was set aside in the bank and by the end of a year formed a substantial portion of the cost of a most enjoyable vacation in my home country. Recollections of this particular vacation were interwoven with pleasant thoughts of appreciation of the patient whose very existence seemed to have made it possible. Although this is a somewhat abstract representation of a need, once recognized, it was not difficult to appreciate that it represented something quite primitive, which might be compared with the need of the nursing mother for her child. The therapist must be prepared to experience something similar to an undifferentiated state of contentment in which he is not motivated to be very active professionally and against which vague boredom and uneasiness act as a defence.

A cardinal feature of this is the urge to be more active, or to give moral advice to oneself to make the right interpretation to hasten the patient's health, rather than to let the time slide rather heedlessly past as it seems to have an uncanny knack of doing.

SCHIZOPHRENIC REACTIONS

In considering schizophrenic reactions, with particular reference to the nature of the transference to the therapist, it is important to appreciate that the phenomenon of regression is a marked feature of the mental processes. Although the core of the psychology of such patients is narcissistic, and the nature of the object choice as primitive as that of an autistic individual, this second group of factors (regressive) tends to obscure the basic nature of the transference. Although it is true that the non-psychotic aspect of the ego functions acts as the ally of the therapist, particularly through the collaboration of its self-reflective capacity, the therapist should not lose sight of the fact that the basic transference is similar to that described in the preceding section. Just as the transference neurosis may tend at its peak to overwhelm the ego in the course of the working-through of a neurotic disorder, so the transference psychosis similarly overwhelms that psychic institution (ego) in the course of psycho-analysis or of a treatment based on psychoanalytic principles. There is a difference, however, and that is that, with the weakened ego structure, the ego tends to be overwhelmed earlier and for longer periods than is the case in the neuroses.

It is on this account that Paul Federn, the earliest worker in this field, recommended that the analyst should discontinue therapy and place the patient in the care of a mothering figure when the negative transference emerged. It was his view that treatment should be suspended until the transference subsided, because he felt that the flooding of the ego with destructive impulses would do irreparable damage. Although he did not spell it out so clearly, it would appear that he felt similarly toward the flooding of the ego with libidinal impulses, for he at one point speculates seriously on the usefulness of castration to prevent such a development.

However one may view these recommendations, it is a fact that the emergence into awareness of strong drives that are highly differentiated can at times make treatment extremely difficult, since the patient often suffers, as a result of structural deficiencies, from a marked lack of impulse control. In this sense, the residues of differentiated mental

P

activity are no ally to the therapist and can in fact be a major factor in an unsuccessful outcome of treatment. In a similar way, the affects are more sharply refined and one runs into acute panic states, feelings of the uncanny, and the other phenomena described by Sullivan (1932), which in the clinical situation are much more disruptive than the kind of organismic distress already described in autism.

In my experience narcissistic somatization of the psychotic process is the most marked feature of catatonia. The entire conflict is enacted physically. The statement that the catatonic develops waxy flexibility as a defence against the destruction of the world is true if one thinks of the world in a Kantian sense, but one must not assume that this factor is involved in such a state. One patient with whom I worked had been mute for seventeen years. When he finally began to speak he said, 'If I talk, my father will have a fit.' The patient experienced this statement of his concretely, and felt that his father would die. It was nonetheless true, however, that in the modern slang sense of the expression his father certainly would have had a fit if he had heard what his son had to say. For example, he declined to acknowledge or recognize his parents' regular weekly visits throughout twenty-three years of mental-hospital life. When he had begun to talk, albeit to a limited extent, to the staff, he was asked one day by a nurse if he knew who the elderly couple were. The nurse finally said, 'That man was your father,' and the patient responded, 'So that's who that old bastard is who brings me orange juice every Saturday.'

Another catatonic patient was assaultive and this feature, of course, rapidly became part of his relationship with the therapist. It is not part of my therapeutic plan to be the object of such attentions, and his reactions, physical and verbal, were energetic. In response to this, the patient used to say, 'Thank you,' but would not elaborate on this response, which always puzzled me, until an occasion when the father visited. He was a physician himself. In the course of his visit, he was struck violently in the mouth by the patient and sustained injuries that required several sutures. When he was asked afterwards what he had done when treated in this way, he stated that he felt that he had behaved in a proper and 'physicianly' manner in that he had understood that the blow was a manifestation of his son's illness. At this point it was clear thatt he patient's 'thank you' was a discriminated response demonstrating that he appreciated the difference between his therapist and his father whose 'physicianly' attitude undoubtedly had emotional significance. The most important point in the story rests on the fact that the catatonic defence had components derived from the father which were not part of early oral narcissism. These factors were subsequently verified in the course of the work as it became clear that the patient had carried into his relationship with his father unsatisfied needs from his early relationship with his mother.

These features were enacted most violently in the early phases of treatment, for the patient succeeded in entering a phase of 'extremis' so intense that the therapist had to intervene in a medical role. When dehydrated, the patient either would not or could not imbibe any fluids of any sort and even when tube-fed he invariably regurgitated the tube-feed. Attempts to sedate him for venous infusion were similarly unsuccessful. However, he invariably swallowed and retained those fluids forced upon him by the therapist, who was thus cast in a quite special role, as a kind of medical saviour. During this period, his thought content was of some interest, for he regarded himself as Jesus Christ, who was suffering to protect the world. When this defence had been dealt with, the patient finally revealed that he felt that his family was afflicted with cruel insanity and that if he suffered in a mental hospital the rest of the family would be safe.

During this period of the work, he reported instances of mental disturbance within the family, which had not been available through history-taking with the other family members, but was confirmed subsequently. Like the mute patient, he was unable to appreciate at that time that the role of the scapegoat contains but meanwhile merely perpetuates the family psychopathology. Behind all this highly complex psychopathology, of course, lay the basic transference to the mother and it was only after this initial material had been gone over that I began to hear of 'the bad mother who had poisoned him by bringing him up by the book'. When this material had been worked over and I had had my full share of being treated as a persecutor, the positive aspects of the relationship with the mother began to appear in the transference and accordingly became available for analysis.

The transference nature of the violence in the initial stages became clear subsequently, for in the interactions the therapist was always the winner. After this phase was over, I discovered that the patient was an expert in unarmed combat, judo, and karate, skills which he had kept hidden, but which were the explanation of why three hefty male nurses or one rather slight therapist were required to subdue him. This transference enactment in the therapy certainly tends to build up omnipotent feelings in the therapist, giving him to feel that only he can be useful to the patient in highly dramatic situations such as the one just described. To misinterpret the fact that it is a transference reaction will lead the therapy down the same useless path as the one described with the autistic patient where the therapist's interpretations were always confirmed. The catatonic individual behind the fragmented remnants of more complex psychogenetic structure and differentiated drives and affects has fundamentally the same type of object-relatedness and tries just as hard to ensure the continuation of the narcissistic gratifications which he is seeking from the therapist in this state.

In the course of work with patients suffering from schizophrenia, one soon finds that, although the patient tends to employ the particular defence mechanisms characteristic of the original categories, it is a mistake to assume that a catatonic patient will not at times present predominantly hebephrenic or paranoid features. On the whole, it has been my experience that the hebephrenic represents the most regressed condition, paranoid states the least. Although regression under the pressure of the oral drives is the rule rather than the exception, it need not be total over a period of time, but more often manifests itself in brief flashes during a session. The more total type of regression can be quite disconcerting to the therapist, as I found when an interesting, verbally fluent, paranoid patient regressed into a mute and helpless catatonic state after several months of therapy. A quite useful manoeuvre in the face of such a situation is to give the responsibility to the patient and ask him to explain what he thinks has happened.

With the predominantly hebephrenic group the exchanges tend to remain on a verbal level. As the communications are characterized, however, by word salad and indirect representation, their value as communication power is somewhat dubious at times. Once again, the therapist should be alert, for the temptation to become an expert in the translating of the patient's particular brand of 'schizophrenese' is always great (Burnham, 1955). On one occasion, I was conducting an administrative ward meeting in a unit where this system had just been introduced. A hebephrenic patient began to talk about washing machines, interspersing odd comments on the two major American political parties. I responded by saying, 'It sounds as though you find our new political system rather phony, and object to the washing of dirty linen in public.' The patient responded with great delight and it was only later, when I was more familiar with such patients, that I was able to appreciate that my comment had not been a masterpiece of therapeutic intervention but rather that the patient had responded to my interest in her.

As one works with such patients, one soon begins to grasp the importance of psychic structure. Although the patient may have some concepts of the rules of living, these are loosely cathected (primary process) and consequently disappear under the influence of strong drives and their affects. Quite often in the analytic situation one may make the mistake of spelling out the rules of treatment in the same manner as one would with someone suffering from a neurosis. I do not mean that there is anything wrong with the ordinary rules, but that they contain implicit within them assumptions which may not be made when dealing with disturbed individuals. The therapist should make clear that he does not tolerate physical attacks and smashing of furniture and that he expects the patient merely to sit on a chair or lie on the couch and talk. Such fundamental rules frequently have to be spelled out with patients suffering from any of the narcissistic disorders. In my experience, these patients appreciate incisive instructions in the analytic situation since, within their own being, structure is so markedly lacking.

With patients of paranoid type, ego structure is much more highly developed, although the paranoid distortions often, though not invariably, so involve the ego that the self-reflective capacity is for long periods incapacitated. Once again, the therapist should remember the rules from the management of autistic transference and not rush in too eagerly. The increase in structure in such patients of necessity leads to delay and consequently a greater degree of stability in the maintenance of negative or positive transference reactions. During the positive phase the therapist will find that his interpretations tend to receive a confirmatory reaction from the patient. These responses, within the limits of intelligence, fundamentally lack discrimination to the same extent as in the autistic patient described above. Superficially, it is more difficult to appreciate this fact if one ignores the basic nature of the object-relatedness, which is obscured by a highly complex psychic structuring containing many of the secondary processes of mentation, but is, nonetheless, basically narcissistic.

Unfortunately for therapy, when the transference shifts to a negative position (Olinick, 1964), such patients tend to reject everything they consider was put into them by their therapist. A useful manoeuvre in dealing with such patients is to ensure to the best of one's ability that the discoveries made in the course of the work are made by the patient. For example, when attempting to explore the thought processes of such an individual, one might ask, 'What do you think of the way you are thinking?' After listening to a paranoid elaboration, it is useful to say merely, 'What is the actual evidence you have for your conclusions?' Such a position tends to leave the discoveries to the patient, while at the same time reinforcing his self-reflective awareness. It has been my experience that the paranoid individual in the negative state does not abandon those discoveries which he feels to be his own, and may even, during such a phase, intensify his analytic efforts.

The work done with such patients may frequently last for many years, involving the analysis of complex interpersonal reactions, including sibling rivalry and marital relations. Only much later do the actual narcissistic and symbiotic aspects of the illness become available for analysis. Since one knows by definition that such material is there, one carries through with the work, knowing well that it will have to be reviewed in other and more mature terms when the narcissistic injury has finally been corrected. In the course of one seven-year treatment attempt with a paranoid patient, I found that the paranoid scapegoating which I had studied with the patient during the early period of therapy could be explored in the context of sibling rivalry with entirely different meaning after the symbiotic relationship with the mother had been dealt with in therapy.

In emphasizing the importance of watching for the basic nature of the transference, I do not mean to imply that the therapist listens in a rejecting manner to the patient's communications. For example, one paranoid woman described a delusional system roughly as follows. 'I wish to go to Arabia. By mental telepathy I have established a relationship with an Arabian prince. He lives in the desert and rides on a white horse. He is wise in the eastern philosophies and rules his own people. Why don't you let me out of this hell-hole so that I can go there and be married to him?' The therapist responded, 'Are you telling me that you can only have a lasting relationship with someone who is far, far away, very powerful and very wise?' The patient responded by describing in a half-hour's tirade how, whenever she became attached to a friend, her parents succeeded in disrupting the relationship. The therapist finally asked if she was giving him a warning regarding his relationship with her and she replied, 'Yes, if the treatment goes well, they will interfere.' Despite this warning the prediction proved accurate, for the family did interrupt the treatment, although the therapist had taken cognizance of the fact that the patient was warning him of her own responsibilities, namely, her own feeling that any positive relationship which she developed was fundamentally destructive.

Another aspect of the transference which the therapist working in an institution should never forget and which Freud was at pains to point out, is that the transference is to the institution as a whole. Comments from the patient regarding the institution should be heard, although not necessarily interpreted, as having meaning in that context. In a situation in which the therapist hears himself described as good and wise and the rest of the therapeutic team as evil and stupid, he should be alert to the splitting of the transference which has as its aim, of course, to maintain him in a good and nurturing role. Should the therapist yield to the temptation to fit himself into this omnipotent and omniscient role, the result is a therapeutic failure, which not merely leaves the patient in an unimproved state, but may seriously impair the therapist's working relationship with the rest of the team and so damage his work with other patients as well.

It is not merely in the early stages of the work that one must watch this phenomenon carefully, for, as has already been mentioned, the resolution of the narcissistic and symbiotic difficulties often, or even usually, occurs comparatively late in the work. For example, the patient who wishes to leave the hospital because the place is no good, the administrator too restrictive, or the staff unimaginative, etc., is a patient who is not yet ready for outpatient status, for the patient is someone who has not yet faced up to the value of the 'lousy rules of living'. If one does not wish one's patient to become suddenly aware of the value of the hospital and its administrative structure in the middle of the night, alone in a down-town apartment, one should take care that this aspect of the relationship to the hospital, to the therapist, and consequently to the parental figures in the past, has been adequately analysed. It is a good rule of thumb that the patient should have some differentiated view of the hospital, varying from an awareness of its areas of usefulness on the one hand to an appreciation of where it was not useful on the other, prior to a move to outpatient status.

One of the biggest stumbling-blocks encountered in the analytic management of the transference is the handling of the phenomenon of negativism, a subject which has recently received attention by Olinick (1964). Negativism, of course, is a normal phase of development, manifesting itself soon after the first appearance of ambivalence. When it originally emerges, this negativism appears as the 'affirmative no' which, in the relationship with the mother, is the first expression of separateness. When the phenomenon appears in the transference of a patient emerging from orality, the difficulty for the therapist is compounded by the presence of regressive factors. However, even with an autistic patient, the therapy with the therapist with whom the work started may be interrupted. One autistic patient with whom the author worked had successfully passed through some useful ambivalent experiences. He came in one day looking pleased, a little surprised, and much more like a person than he ever had done before. He said, 'I've just discovered something. I didn't pick you for my doctor. My mother did. You're fired. I'm going to get a doctor of my own.' He carried through this intention.

With patients in the schizophrenic category, however, negativism is both more obscure and more apt to be highly disruptive. It requires to be differentiated from the genuine negative transference (see Chapter 3). Nonetheless, it closely resembles a negative transference and the patient may experience the reaction as a wish to destroy the therapist. Behind the angry and threatening demeanour lies the same need to be a separate individual as appears in a child's affirmative no (A. Freud, 1951). It has seemed to me for some time, and in this I am in agreement with Olinick, that both the malevolent transformation and the negative therapeutic reaction are pathological derivatives of this period of early psychogenesis. It is not infrequent, for example, for the patient to become particularly difficult, abusive, or even violent, when he feels that he is apt to be engulfed because of his positive feelings towards the therapist. This kind of reaction is well documented in a paper by Jacobson (1954).

DEPRESSIVE REACTIONS

The narcissistic depressive reactions have as their fixation point a psychogenetically later phase of orality than do the schizophrenic reactions. The patient's mentation is characterized by a greater degree of structure, and the introjects are much more highly differentiated and stable. This tends to alter the nature of the object-relatedness in the transference, and it is characterized by a much greater degree of specificity, though it should not be forgotten that fundamentally the relationship is still oral. The depressive factor operates as a constant alertness on the part of the patient to the possibility that he will damage his therapist. Beyond that again, however, lies the firmly held belief that, should he allow his destructiveness to operate in destroying his therapist, he will destroy himself, since he is totally dependent on him as a particular individual for his very survival. Quite often this constant anxiety leads to an extraordinary sensitivity to the emotional and physical well-being of the therapist.

The accuracy of these observations should not obscure the therapist's awareness of the terrifying, narcissistic use which the patient makes of such observations. One day I was interviewing a woman who had such difficulties. I had wakened that morning feeling slightly out of sorts and suffering from a mild headache. The patient kept looking at me throughout the session, stealing quick and frightened glances and commenting that I did not seem in good form. She was convinced that she had said something the previous day. Attempts at exploring this failed during the hour in question. The patient's repeated comments, however, did direct my attention to the fact that I was not merely unusually heavy that morning, but was in fact much more out of sorts than I had realized. When I checked my temperature subsequently, it was nearly 103° F. and it became clear that I was in the early stages of an attack of Asian flu. As the work with this woman progressed, I discovered clear evidence that during her very early childhood, she had been nursed by a depressed mother who had required much active demonstration of affection from her children to reassure her low self-esteem. In order to get to the point of this realization, of course, manifestations of this particular depressive position had had to appear and be worked through repetitiously in the transference. The amount of energy cathected in this situation should never be underestimated, despite the masking of its movement by complex secondary processes.

Relaxation of careful administration may lead to a violent, self-destructive act at the very moment of analytic success. Work with one such patient ended particularly sadly, as follows. The patient, a fifty-four-year-old manic-depressive woman, who had been quite ill for the best part of twenty-five years, had been working very satisfactorily with me for three years. She was working actively on the depressive-narcissistic nucleus mentioned above. Following the successful trans-ference analysis of these components, the patient began one day to talk about her mother. She drew together quickly in summary form many factors previously described. She returned again to an incident in her middle teens which had always seemed of some particular importance to her. She had gone to a teenage party wearing a dress especially made for her by her mother. For her the party had been a flop, and she felt like a wall-flower. On her return home she had told her mother that things had been all right. She had then gone to her bed and wept into her pillow, sleeplessly.

On previously occasions she had examined mainly her deviousness, her secretiveness, or some other quality which had appeared in the transference. On this occasion she saw it in a different light, saying angrily, 'How the hell, doctor, could I tell her of my unhappiness and my pain. I could not tell her that I felt I was a flop and a failure. She could not have tolerated that, because she would have felt that it was somehow her failure and I would have had to spend the rest of the night consoling her and ignoring what I myself was feeling. I have spent all my life feeling that I was dependent on her. The truth of the matter is that she, the bitch, was so dependent on me that my needs were never met. God damn it! That's what has kept me a dependent person all my life.' When she left the office, flushed and angry, I thought that the patient was well on her way towards the resolution of a severe and protracted illness. That night, unfortunately, the patient died of a sub-arachnoid haemorrhage from an aneurism of the circle of Willis. There is no doubt in my mind that the rise in her blood-pressure associated with the affective storm resulting from the resolution of the depressive nucleus was at the least an important contributory factor to her death at that point.

In the behavioural sense, the difference between mania and depression is a marked one. However, in the course of working intensively with persons suffering from these conditions over prolonged periods, one becomes less inclined to make such a sharp differentiation between the psychological processes involved in the two states. In addition, one usually has to revise one's preconceived notions about the affective tone of the two states. For example, I regard the depressive state as being a much more angry one than is the maniacal condition. Freud's comment that the manic patient seeks object-relations as a starving man seeks bread, describes the core of this, for the maniacal individual is terrified, alone, despairing, and convinced that he has destroyed all his objects. The tremendous rush of speech serves, not as communication, but as a hedge of spears which one cannot penetrate. Working with the depressed patient, one encounters the identical hedge.

It has been my experience that, in the early phases of treatment, attention is best directed predominantly to fairly simple comments regarding the over-critical superego functions. During this period, one sees clearly not merely the constant expectation of criticism through the projection of the superego role onto the therapist, but also the constant expectation already mentioned, namely that some kind of damage will befall the therapist. With patients in this group, the manifestations of negativism are particularly important. For example, one of my patients, a woman who had been ill for a number of years, alternated between a tremendously disturbed maniacal state and a silent and non-responsive condition, so that one could not be sure that she was even depressed and despairing. Fairly typical of her behaviour during such periods was the following exchange during a session. When asked the standard analytic question, 'What comes to mind?' she would not respond for a minute or so. She would shake her head and respond, 'A blank'. 'What comes to mind about a blank?' Again the shake of the head and the answer, 'Nothing'.

After some fourteen months of work, this particular aspect of the relationship became the focal point of treatment and I interpreted her persistent saying of 'no' as a resistance to treatment. The data that emerged following this were particularly interesting, for she revealed, in a multiplicity of ways, how she used to say 'no' to her mother. One way, after her marriage, was simply not to see her mother, and avoid visiting her or having her mother visit her home. Following her father's death, she felt an obligation to have her mother stay with her for a month. From the patient's point of view, the visit was an absolute nightmare involving an enactment of the worst fears of her childhood, for the mother, distraught with grief and distress from an abnormal mourning, was too totally preoccupied with herself to accept her daughter's attempts to comfort her and failed completely to recognize that her daughter, too, was in mourning.

In this state, her behaviour towards her daughter was practically a caricature of the over-anxious, nagging, and perfectionistic upbringing to which she had subjected her. A month or two later, at the urging of her two brothers, the patient went off to visit her mother in a state many miles away. On her arrival, she was found to be for the first time in the acute state of mania, which from then onwards led to her frequent hospitalizations. The identifications that complicated the negativism were of considerable interest also. Her father, who was a somewhat silent individual, had a typical way of dealing with the emotionality of his wife. When things became too difficult for him, he would simply get up and walk silently out of the house, returning equally silently when he felt he had given his wife enough time to cool down. The patient's comment about this is interesting. 'But I was a child, so I couldn't walk out. I tried to be as good as I could, but even perfection was no protection, so I had to find ways of my own to say no, in order to survive.' Of course, this aspect of the introjected father had a great deal to do with her fear of her own emotions, and acted as a powerful reinforcement for the fundamental depressive position of the earlier psychogenetic phase.

Another theme in this woman's treatment was the fear of being defective. She gave a great deal of evidence to support the view that there was something neurologically wrong with her family in the hereditary sense. Her only child had been hydrocephalic and she spoke of the vagueness surrounding the deaths of some of her relatives when she was a child. Her mania was characterized by behaviour that was remarkably idiotic and foolish. It reminded me of what an intelligent but non-professional person would expect an idiot to do under stress. Exploration of this led to the discovery that she was profoundly convinced that someone as inept as she basically felt she was must be defective, neurologically. If it was not that *she* was an idiot, then her mother must be. And if her mother was, then by heredity, so was she.

One feature of this aspect of the work with the patient in a maniacal phase is that even when one is not able to interrupt a maniacal process, one must nonetheless remain working on the same fixed schedule as before, observing the patient's state extremely carefully. Such a state can be viewed as a frantic enactment of, a desperate restitutive attempt to deal with, the patient's most profound fears. The patient being described, for example, expressed and enacted the entire depressive nucleus of her illness, including her conviction in fragmented, delusional form, that she had destroyed her husband, her two sons, and her therapist. The latter's steadfast refusal to be dead, by continuing to see her at the same time daily, she afterwards stated, had been particularly comforting to her during those terrifying episodes, of which she and the therapist survived six during their work.

SUMMARY

In this chapter I have attempted to follow one particular theme regarding the analytic treatment of psychotic states, namely, some considerations on the nature of the transference. Proposing that the clinical state of autism should be regarded as a somewhat approximate equivalent to pure orality, I have attempted, in extremely summarized form, to demonstrate the increasing complexity which occurs through later psychogenetic influences. In the section dealing with depression and mania, for example, no direct reference has been made at all to the important and ever-present mechanism of denial. Many other equally important processes in all clinical categories have been ignored for the purposes of brevity.

If one follows the classical theory by paying attention to an oedipus complex, then one must pay attention to the existence of the narcissistic oedipus complex, narcissistic reversed oedipal states, narcissistic urethral and anal manifestations, and other examples of conflicts and structure. These mental conditions of unstable equilibrium, as has been indicated, masquerade as being similar to their non-narcissistic equivalent. The analyst of narcissistic states remains cognizant of this fact as he pursues his patient's health through the careful and methodical analysis of the basic oral trauma.

Bibliography

ABRAHAM, K. (1913). Restrictions and transformations of scopophilia. *Selected papers*. London: Hogarth Press, 1942.

ADRIAN, E. D. (1946). The mental and physical origins of behaviour. Ernest Jones Lecture. *Int. J. Psycho-Anal.*, **27**, 1.

ANGYAL, A. (1936). The experience of the body self in schizophrenia. *Arch. Neurol. & Psychiat.*, **35**, 1029.

BATCHELOR, I. R. C. (1964). The diagnosis of schizophrenia. *Proc. Roy. Soc. Med.*, **57**, 417.

BION, W. R. (1957). Differentiation of the psychotic from the non-psychotic personalities. *Int. J. Psycho-Anal.*, **38**, 266.

BION, W. R. (1958). On hallucination. *Int. J. Psycho-Anal.*, **39**, 341.

BION, W. R. (1959). Attacks on linking. *Int. J. Psycho-Anal.*, **40**, 308.

BLEULER, E. (1911). *Dementia praecox or the group of schizophrenias*. New York: International Universities Press.

BLEULER, M. (1963). Conception of schizophrenia within the last fifty years and today. *Proc. Roy. Soc. Med.*, **56**, 945.

BOWLBY, J. (1960). Separation anxiety. *Int. J. Psycho-Anal.*, **41**, 89.

BRAIN, R. (1958). The physiological basis of consciousness. *Brain*, **81**, 426.

BROADBENT, D. E. (1958). *Perception and communication*. London: Pergamon Press.

BURNHAM, D. L. (1955). Some problems in communication with schizophrenic patients. *J. Amer. Psychoanal. Assoc.*, **3**, 67.

BYCHOWSKI, G. (1943). Disturbance of the body image in the clinical picture of psychosis. *J. Nerv. Ment. Dis.*, **97**, 310.

CAMERON, J. L. (1963). Patient, therapist, and administrator: a study of a conflictual situation. *Brit. J. Med. Psychol.*, **36**, 13.

CAMERON, N. (1961). Introjection, reprojection and hallucination in the interaction between schizophrenic patient and therapist. *Int. J. Psycho-Anal.*, **42**, 86.

CHAPMAN, J., FREEMAN, T., and MCGHIE, A. (1959). Clinical research in schizophrenia. *Brit. J. Med. Psychol.*, **32**, 75.

CHAPMAN, J. and MCGHIE, A. (1962). A comparative study of disordered attention in schizophrenia. *J. Ment. Sci.*, **108**, 455, 487.

CONRAD, R. (1964). Acoustic confusions in immediate memory. *Brit. J. Psychol.*, **55**, 1, 75–84.

CRITCHLEY, M. (1951). Discussion on parietal lobe syndromes. *Proc. Roy. Soc. Med.*, **44**, 337.

CRITCHLEY, M. (1953). *The parietal lobes*. London: Arnold.

CURRAN, F. J. and SCHILDER, P. (1935). Paraphasic signs in diffuse lesions of the brain. *J. Nerv. Ment. Dis.*, **82**, 613.

DARR, G. C. and WORDEN, F. G. (1951). Case report: twenty-eight years after an infantile autistic disorder. *Amer. J. Orthopsychiatry*, **21**, 3, 559.

DAVIE, J. M. (1963). Observations on some defensive aspects of delusion formation. *Brit. J. Med. Psychol.*, **36**, 67.

DAVIE, J. M. and FREEMAN, T. (1961). The non-psychotic residue in schizophrenia. *Brit. J. Med. Psychol.*, **34**, 117.

FAIRBAIRN, W. R. D. (1952). *Psycho-analytic studies of the personality*. London: Tavistock Publications.

FARBER, LESLIE H. (1958). The therapeutic despair. *Psychiatry*, **21**, 1, 7.

FARBER, LESLIE H. (1963). Schizophrenia and the mad psychotherapist. *J. Exist. Psychol. & Psychiat.*, **3**, 3, 209.

FEDERN, P. (1943). Psycho-analysis of psychoses. In P. FEDERN (Ed.), *Ego psychology and the psychoses*, 1953.

FEDERN, P. (1948). Mental hygiene of the ego in schizophrenia. In P. FEDERN (Ed.), *Ego psychology and the psychoses*, 1953.

FEDERN, P. (1949). The ego in schizophrenia. In P. FEDERN (Ed.), *Ego psychology and the psychoses*, 1953.

FEDERN, P. (1953). *Ego psychology and the psychoses*. London: Imago; New York: Basic Books.

FERSTER, C. B. (1961). Positive reinforcement and behavioral deficits of autistic children. *Child Development*, **32**, 437.

FISHER, C. (1956). Dreams, images and perception. *J. Amer. Psychoanal. Assoc.*, **4**, 5.

FRAZER, J. G. (1890). *The golden bough*. London & New York: Macmillan.

FREEMAN, T. (1958). The contribution of psychoanalysis to the problem of schizophrenia. In T. F. RODGER, R. M. MOWBRAY, and J. R. ROY (Eds.), *Topics in psychiatry*. London: Cassell.

FREEMAN, T. (1962). Psycho-analytic observation of chronic schizophrenic reactions. In J. M. TANNER (Ed.), *Aspects of psychiatric research*. London: Oxford University Press.

FREEMAN, T. (1962a). A psycho-analytic approach to the diagnosis of schizophrenic reactions. *J. Ment. Sci.*, **108**.

FREEMAN, T. (1962b). Narcissism and defensive processes in schizophrenic reactions. *Int. J. Psycho-Anal.*, **43**, 415.

FREEMAN, T. (1963). The concept of narcissism in schizophrenic states. *Int. J. Psycho-Anal.*, **44**, 293.

FREEMAN, T. (1964). Aspects of pathological narcissism. *J. Amer. Psychoanal. Assoc.*, **12**, 540.

FREEMAN, T., CAMERON, J. L. and MCGHIE, A. (1958). *Chronic schizophrenia.* London: Tavistock Publications; New York: International Universities Press.

FREEMAN, T. and MCGHIE, A. (1957). The relevance of genetic psychology for the psycho-pathology of schizophrenia. *Brit. J. Med. Psychol.*, **30**, 176.

FRENKEL-BRUNSWIK, E. (1951). In R. BLAKE and A. V. RAMSAY (Eds.), *Perception: an approach to personality.* New York: Ronald Press.

FREUD, A. (1936). *The ego and the mechanisms of defence.* London: Hogarth Press, 1948; New York: International Universities Press.

FREUD, A. (1951). A connection between the states of negativism and emotional surrender. *Int. J. Psycho-Anal.*, **32**, 265.

FREUD, A. (1952). Mutual influences in the development of ego and id. *Psychoanalytic study of the child*, **7**, 18. London: Imago; New York: International Universities Press.

FREUD, S. (1900). *The interpretation of dreams.* London: Allen & Unwin, 1955; New York: Basic Books.

FREUD, S. (1909). Family romances. *Collected Papers*, **5**, 74. London: Hogarth Press, 1950.

FREUD, S. (1911). Psycho-analytic notes upon an autobiographical account of a case of paranoia. *Collected papers*, **3**, 387. London: Hogarth Press, 1925.

FREUD, S. (1914). On narcissism: an introduction. *Collected papers*, **4**, 30. London: Hogarth Press, 1947.

FREUD, S. (1915). The unconscious. *Collected papers*, **4**, 98. London: Hogarth Press, 1947.

FREUD, S. (1916). Metapsychological supplement to the theory of dreams. *Collected papers*, **4**, 137. London: Hogarth Press, 1947.

FREUD, S. (1917). Mourning and melancholia. *Collected papers*, **4**, 152. London: Hogarth Press, 1947.

FREUD, S. (1923). *The ego and the id.* London: Hogarth Press, 1947.

FREUD, S. (1924). Neurosis and psychosis. *Collected papers*, **2**, 250. London: Hogarth Press, 1947.

FREUD, S. (1937). Analysis terminable and interminable. *Collected papers*, **5**, 316. London: Hogarth Press, 1950.

FROSCH, J. (1960). An examination of nosology according to psychoanalytic concepts. *J. Amer. Psychoanal. Assoc.*, **8**, 535.

GARDINER, R. W. (1962). *The development of cognitive structures.* Memorial Meeting, University of Kansas.

GELLHORN, E. and LOOFBOURROW, G. N. (1963). *Emotions and emotional disorder.* New York: Hoeber.

GILLESPIE, W. H. (1963). Some regressive phenomena in old age. *Brit. J. Med. Psychol.*, **36**, 203.

Q

GLOVER, E. (1932). A psycho-analytical approach to the classification of mental disorders. In E. GLOVER (Ed.), *On the early development of mind*. London: Imago, 1956; New York: International Universities Press.

GLOVER, E. (1954). The indications for psycho-analysis. In E. GLOVER (Ed.), *On the early development of mind*. London: Imago, 1956; New York: International Universities Press.

GLOVER, E. (1955). *The technique of psycho-analysis*. London: Baillière, Tindall & Cox; New York: International Universities Press.

GLOVER, E. (1964). Research techniques in psycho-analysis and in general psychology: an essay in contrasts. In J. COHEN (Ed.), *Readings in Psychology*. London: Allen & Unwin.

HARTMANN, H. (1939). *Ego psychology and the problem of adaptation*. London: Imago, 1958; New York: International Universities Press.

HARTMANN, H. (1951). Ego psychology and the problem of adaptation. In D. RAPAPORT (Ed.), *Organization and pathology of thought*. New York: Columbia University Press.

HARTMANN, H. (1952). Mutual influences in development of ego and id. *Psycho-analytic study of the child*, **7**. London: Imago; New York: International Universities Press.

HARTMANN, H. (1953). Contribution to the metapsychology of schizophrenia. *Psycho-analytic study of the child*, **8**, 177. London: Imago; New York: International Universities Press.

HAVENS, L. L. (1962). Replacement and movement of hallucinations in space: phenomenology and theory. *Int. J. Psycho-Anal.*, **43**, 426.

HERDAN, G. (1958). The statistical interpretation of aphasia. *Confin. Psychiat.*, **1**, 143.

HILGARD, E. R. (1951). In R. BLAKE and G. V. RAMSAY (Eds.), *Perception: an approach to personality*. New York: Ronald Press.

HILL, D. (1962). The schizophrenia-like psychoses of epilepsy. *Proc. Roy. Soc. Med.*, **55**, 315.

HOFFER, W. (1954). Defensive process and defensive organisation. *Int. J. Psycho-Anal.*, **35**, 194.

HOLT, R. R. (1962). A critical reassessment of Freud's concept of bound vs. free cathexis. *J. Amer. Psychoanal. Assoc.*, **10**, 475.

HOLZMAN, P. S. (1954). The relation of assimilation tendencies in visual, auditory and kinaesthetic time error to cognitive attitudes of levelling and sharpening. *J. Personality*, **22**, 315.

JACOBSON, E. (1954). On psychotic identifications. *Int. J. Psycho-Anal.*, **35**, 102.

JACOBSON, E. (1954a). The self and the object world. *Psycho-analytic study of the child*, **9**. London: Imago; New York: International Universities Press.

JONES, E. (1953). *Sigmund Freud – life and work*, **1**. London: Hogarth Press; New York: Basic Books.

JUNG, C. G. (1907). The psychology of dementia praecox. *Coll. works*, **3**, London: Routledge & Kegan Paul, 1960.

KANNER, L. (1949). Problems of nosology and psychodynamics of early infantile autism. *Amer. J. Orthopsychiatry*, **19**, 416.

KATAN, M. (1950). Structural aspects of a case of schizophrenia. *Psycho-analytic study of the child*, **5**. London: Imago; New York: International Universities Press.

KATAN, M. (1954). The non-psychotic part of the personality in schizophrenia. *Int. J. Psycho-Anal.*, **35**, 119.

KETY, S. (1961). The heuristic aspect of psychiatry. *Amer. J. Psychiat.*, **118**, 385.

KING, G. F. and RABIN, A. I. (1959). Psychological studies. In L. BELLAK (ed.), *Schizophrenia — a review of the syndrome*. New York: Logos Press.

KLEIN, G. S. (1954). Need and regulation. In M. R. JONES (Ed.), *Nebraska symposium on motivation*. Lincoln, Nebr.: Nebraska University Press.

KLEIN, G. S. (1959). Consciousness in psychoanalytic theory — some implications for current research in perception. *J. Amer. Psychoanal. Assoc.*, **7**, 5.

LAFFAL, J. (1961). Changes in the language of a schizophrenic patient during psychotherapy. *J. Abnorm. & Soc. Psychol.*, **63**, 422.

LAWSON, J. S., MCGHIE, A. and CHAPMAN, J. (1964). Perception of speech in schizophrenia. *Brit. J. Psychiat.*, **110**, 375.

LINDSLEY, B. (1960). Attention, consciousness, sleep and wakefulness. In *Handbook of Physiology*, section 1, Neurophysiology, **3**. Baltimore: Williams & Wilkins.

MCGHIE, A. and CHAPMAN, J. (1961). Disorders of attention and perception in early schizophrenia. *Brit. J. Med. Psychol.*, **34**, 103.

MCGHIE, A., CHAPMAN, J. and LAWSON, J. S. (1965). The effect of distraction on schizophrenic performance — (1) Perception and immediate memory. *Brit. J. Psychiat.*, **111**, 383.

MCGHIE, A., CHAPMAN, J. and LAWSON, J. S. (1965a). Changes in immediate memory with age. *Brit. J. Psychol.*, **56**, 1.

MCGHIE, A., CHAPMAN, J. and LAWSON, J. S. (1965b). The effect of distraction on schizophrenic performance — psychomotor ability. *Brit. J. Psychiat.*, **111**, 391.

MAHLER, M. (1952). On child psychosis and schizophrenia. *Psycho-analytic study of the child*, **7**, 286. London: Imago; New York: International Universities Press.

MAHLER, M. (1958). Autism and symbiosis. *Int. J. Psycho-Anal.*, **39**, 77.

MAIN, T. F. (1957). The ailment. *Brit. J. Med. Psychol.*, **30**, 129.

MILLER, G. A. and SELFRIDGE, J. A. (1950). Verbal context and the recall of meaningful material. *Amer. J. Psychol.*, **63**, 176.

MILLER, J. G. (1951). In R. BLAKE and G. V. RAMSAY (Eds.), *Perception, an approach to personality*. New York: Ronald Press.

MODELL, H. A. (1958). Hallucinatory experiences in schizophrenia. *J. Amer. Psychoanal. Assoc.*, **6**, 442.

NIEDERLAND, W. G. (1959). The 'miracled up' world of Schreber's childhood. *Psycho-analytic study of the child*, **14**, 383. London: Imago; New York: International Universities Press.

OLINICK, S. L. (1964). The negative therapeutic reaction. *Int. J. Psycho-Anal.*, **45**, 540.

OSTOW, M. (1962). *Drugs in psycho-analysis and psychotherapy.* New York: Basic Books.

PAYNE, R. W. (1961). Cognitive abnormalities. In H. J. EYSENCK (Ed.), *Handbook of abnormal psychology*. New York: Basic Books.

PAYNE, R. W., ANCEVICH, S. and LAVERTY, S. G. (1963). Overinclusive thinking in sympton-free schizophrenics. *Can. Psychiat. Assoc. J.*, **8**, 225.

PAYNE, R. W. and HEWLETT, J. H. G. (1960). Thought disorder in psychotic patients. In H. J. EYSENCK (Ed.), *Experiments in personality*, **2**. London: Routledge & Kegan Paul.

PAYNE, R. W., MATUSSEK, P. and GEORGE, E. I. (1959). An experimental study of schizophrenic thought disorder. *J. Ment. Sci.*, **105**, 627.

PIAGET, J. (1932). *The language and thought of the child.* London: Routledge & Kegan Paul.

PIAGET, J. (1947). *The psychology of intelligence.* London: Routledge & Kegan Paul.

POLLIN, W. (1962). Control and artifact in psychophysiological research. In R. ROESSLER and N. S. GREENFIELD (Eds.), *Psychophysiological correlates of psychological disorder*. Madison: University of Wisconsin Press.

POLLIN, W. and GOLDIN, S. (1962). The physiological and psychological effects of intravenously administered epinephrine and its metabolism in normal and schizophrenic men. *J. Psychiat. Research*, **1**, 24.

RAPAPORT, D. (1951). *Organization and pathology of thought.* New York: Columbia University Press.

RAPAPORT, D. (1953). On the psycho-analytic theory of affects. *Int. J. Psycho-Anal.*, **34**, 117.

RICKMAN, J. (1948). The application of psycho-analytical principles to hospital in-patients. *J. Ment. Sci.*, **94**, 764.

ROSEN, V. H. (1953). On mathematical 'illumination' and the mathematical thought process: a contribution to the genetic development and metapsychology of abstract thinking. *Psycho-analytic study of the child*, **8**, 127. London: Imago; New York: International Universities Press.

ROSENFELD, H. (1952). Transference phenomena and transference analysis in an acute catatonic schizophrenic patient. *Int. J. Psycho-Anal.*, **33**, 451.

SABSHIN, M., HAMBURG, D. A., GRINKER, R. A. *et al.* (1957). Significance of pre-experimental studies in the psychosomatic laboratory. *AMA Arch. Neurol. & Psychiat.*, **78**, 207.

SCHACHTEL, E. G. (1954). The development of focal attention and the emergence of reality. *Psychiat.*, **17**.

SCHILDER, P. (1923). *Medical psychology.* New York: International Universities Press, 1953.

SCHILDER, P. (1928). Akinetic states, stupor and negativism. *Brain and personality.* New York: International Universities Press, 1951.

SCHILDER, P. (1928a). On encephalitis. *Brain and personality.* New York: International Universities Press, 1951.

SCHILDER, P. (1928b). Speech disturbances. *Brain and personality.* New York: International Universities Press, 1951.

SCHILDER, P. (1950). *The image and appearance of the human body.* New York: International Universities Press.

SEARLES, H. F. (1959). The effort to drive the other person crazy — an element in the aetiology and psychotherapy of schizophrenia. *Brit. J. Med. Psychol.*, **32**, 1.

SEARLES, H. F. (1959a). Integration and differentiation in schizophrenia. *Brit. J. Med. Psychol.*, **32**, 261.

SEARLES, H. F. (1960). *The nonhuman environment.* New York: International Universities Press.

SEARLES, H. F. (1961). The evolution of the mother transference in psychotherapy of the psychoses. In BURTON, A. (Ed.), *Psychotherapy of Psychoses.* New York: Basic Books.

SEARLES, H. F. (1961a). Sources of the anxiety in paranoid schizophrenia. *Brit. J. Med. Psychol.*, **34**, 129.

SEARLES, H. F. (1961b) Anxiety concerning change as seen in the psychotherapy of schizophrenic patients. *Int. J. Psycho-Anal.*, **42**, 74.

SEARLES, H. F. (1963). Formal discussion. *Brit. J. Med. Psychol.*, **36**, 22.

SEARLES, H. F. (1963a). Transference psychosis in the psychotherapy of chronic schizophrenia. *Int. J. Psycho-Anal.*, **44**, 249.

SHAKOW, D. (1962). Segmental set. *Arch. Gen. Psychiat.*, **6**, 1.

SHAKOW, D. (1963). Psychological deficit in schizophrenia. *Behav. Sci.*, **8**, 4, 275.

SHANNON, C. E. (1948). A mathematical theory of communication. *Bell Syst. Tech. J.*, **27**, 379.

SHANNON, C. E. (1951). Prediction and entropy of printed English. *Bell Syst. Tech. J.*, **30**, 50.

SLATER, E. and BEARD, A. W. (1963). The schizophrenia-like psychoses of epilepsy. *Brit. J. Psychiat.*, **109**, 95.

SPERLING, G. (1960). The information available in brief visual presentations. *Psychol. Monogr.*, **74**, 11.

STENGEL, E. (1954). The origins and status of dynamic psychiatry. *Brit. J. Med. Psychol.*, **27**, 193.

SULLIVAN, H. S. (1932). The modified psycho-analytic treatment of schizo-phrenia. *Amer. J. Psychiat.*, **88**, 519.

SULLIVAN, H. S. (1962). *Schizophrenia as a human process.* New York: Norton.

SZEKELY, L. (1954). Biological remarks on fears originating in early childhood. *Int. J. Psycho-Anal.*, **35**, 57.

TAIT, A. C. (1958). The physiopathology of schizophrenia. In T. F. RODGER, R. M. MOWBRAY and J. R. ROY (Eds.), *Topics in psychiatry*. London: Cassell.

TAUSK, V. (1919). On the origins of the influencing machine in schizophrenia. *Psychoanal. Quart.*, 1933, **2**, 263.

TIZARD, M. and MARGERISON, J. H. (1963). The relationship between general-ized paroxysmal EEG discharges and various test situations in two epileptic patients. *J. Neurol. Neurosurg. & Psychiat.*, **26**, 308.

VENABLES, P. H. (1963). Selectivity of attention, withdrawal, and cortical acti-vation. *Arch. Gen. Psychiat.*, **9**, 74.

VENABLES, P. H. and O'CONNOR, N. (1959). A short scale for rating paranoid schizophrenia. *J. Ment. Sci.*, **105**, 815.

VENABLES, P. H. and WING, J. K. (1962). Level of arousal and the sub-classifica-tion of schizophrenia. *Arch. Gen. Psychiat.*, **7**, 114.

WECKOWICZ, T. E. and BLEWETT, D. B. (1959). Size constancy and abstract thinking in schizophrenic patients. *J. Ment. Sci.*, **105**, 909.

WEINSTEIN, E. A. and KAHN, R. L. (1950). The syndrome of anosognosia. *Arch. Neurol. & Psychiat.*, **64**, 772.

WERNER, R. (1948). *Comparative psychology of mental development.* New York: International Universities Press.

WINDER, C. L. (1961). Some psychological studies of schizophrenics. In DON D. JACKSON (Ed.), *The aetiology of schizophrenia.* New York: Basic Books.

ZANGWILL, O. (1964). Physiological and experimental psychology. In J. COHEN (Ed.), *Readings in psychology.* London: Allen & Unwin.

Index

Abraham, K., 86
accommodation, 12
acting-out in transference, 121, 139f, 147
adaptation: hallucinations and, 127f; to environment, 88
administration, and therapy, relation, 199ff
Adrian, E. D., 77
adualism, 22, 188
affects(s): flattening of, 3; and physical hyperactivity, 156; in schizophrenia, 35; 'taming' of, 36
affect theory, in psychosis, 34ff
affectivity, 155ff
affirmative no, 215, 223, 224
agrammatism, 105
aim, reversal of, 33, 166, 167, 168
anger: displaced, experiment and, 146f; and reversal of cognitive disorganization, 53
Angyal, A., 162
anosognosia, 168
anxiety: and cognitive dysfunction, 54; and ego regression, 72; projection of, 73
assimilation: of identity, 46f; passive 80; Piaget's concept, 12
attention: as active process, 76; and cognitive functioning, 85f; defects in, 11, 29, 72ff;——, two categories, 81f; disturbance in early schizophrenia, 178ff; model of, 189;

psycho-analytic theory, 75f; selective, 78; theoretical considerations, 81ff
attitude variable, 13, 131
auditory stimuli; falsified perception, 82f; distraction by, and perception, 181; inattention to, 80
autism, 209
auto-erotism, return to, 107

Batchelor, I. R. C., 174
belief, inductive, perversion of, 73, 163
Bell's Mania, 207
biology, and psycho-analysis, 8
Bion, W. R., 27, 28, 29, 131
Bleuler, E., 30, 39, 83, 97, 99
Bleuler, M., 26
block, therapeutic, 206
bodily awareness, disturbances of, 161
Bowlby, J., 8
Brain, R., 189
brain apparatus, and specific functions 53, 169
Broadbent, D. E., 189
Burnham, D. L., 104, 220
Bychowski, G., 161

Cameron, J. L., 125
catatonia, 218
Chapman, J., et al., 161;——, and McGhie, A., 169, 178, 181

239